Politics and Planning in the National Health Service

——— Neil Small

——————— OPEN UNIVERSITY PRESS
——————— MILTON KEYNES · PHILADELPHIA

Open University Press
Celtic Court
22 Ballmoor
Buckingham MK18 1XW

and
1900 Frost Road, Suite 101
Bristol, PA 19007, USA

First Published 1989. Reprinted 1991

British Library Cataloguing in Publication Data

Small, Neil
  Politics and planning in the NHS.
  1. Great Britain. Health services. Political aspects
  I. Title
  362.1'0941

  ISBN 0-335-09264-0
  ISBN 0-335-09259-4 (paper)

Library of Congress Cataloging in Publication Number available

Typeset by Gilbert Composing Services
Printed in Great Britain by
St Edmundsbury Press, Bury St Edmunds, Suffolk

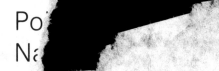
Po   in t
Na   ce

To Horace Small and Mary Small

Contents

Preface

This book is about the National Health Service. Much of the material presented comes from the years 1984 to 1989. These were times when the NHS figured prominently in both public and political discourse. Macaulay said it was not pleasant to live in times about which it was exciting to read (quoted in McLuhan 1964, p. 83) and certainly much of this discourse has concentrated on a sense of these being difficult times – difficult for the patients and potential patients, for the staff of the NHS, for the politicians (and for writers on the NHS who see so many changes that what is written quickly needs modifying in the light of new developments).

Since the Second World War health policy has occupied a central position in the public world of policy-making, just as health care has in the private world of personal experience. Further, it has provided a location for the construction of ideological paradigms about the relationship between the state and the individual and the nature of a caring society. Both the structure of health care delivery and the ideological assumptions that exist alongside it have been subject to considerable scrutiny in recent years. This scrutiny has generated some hope and a lot of fear.

The fear is complex because it addresses the many levels at which the NHS exists for each person. David Owen (1976) remarked that when we are well we are critical of doctors and medicine, when we are sick we want them to be all-knowledgeable. The NHS touches all our lives and figures in our constructions of the future. While I have been writing this work four close members of my family have required considerable medical care. On each occasion the sense of relief that facilities were available was tempered by a recognition that those facilities were in short supply and were sometimes offered with little regard for the patient's being an active participant in the process of treatment and cure. Echoing David Owen, I felt grateful for the skill and sensitivity of the staff; on the other hand, I did not want to be met by an expert who purported to an exclusive knowledgeability.

This personal experience of the NHS will be common to many and because of it the usual language of social policy and political science does not seem sufficient to engage with the subject's private import. The fear generated by NHS reform therefore concerns a feeling that the service we, or those close to us, will need may not be available. It also addresses a sense that a service many of us have grown up with and that we are used to hearing praised as something the United Kingdom can be proud of, our post-Empire example to the world, is being reconstructed or dismantled.

There has not been a tradition of constructively critical debate around health care despite the volumes of print the subject has generated. The NHS, in particular, has been insulated from debate, save around the margins. Issues of funding and organizational structure have dominated and have become the customary debating ground for opposing sides in the politics of health. But what gets missed out in all this struggle is a sense of needs and outputs. Health seems missing in the politics of health.

This work attempts three things. It looks at the structures within which some of the debate on health care is carried on and at the communication of that debate to the outside world. It then looks at some activities that are much discussed in the political and public debate and which appear central to the health care project.

It is my intention to examine the formal and informal, the private and the public, worlds of policy-making in health. To arrive at some sort of understanding of how such worlds interact and generate policy requires identifying a distinction between organizational activity and organizational structure. It is important not just to understand the formal framework for policy-making but to appreciate the way this formal structure interacts with the myriad informal avenues for influence. I will seek to present a description that shows the formal and informal interaction dialectically. They are separate aspects of a unitary process and cannot be presented in some sort of dualistic model. Contradictions will be evident between different parts of the organizational structure and between it and other related structures. There will also be a distinction between activity and outcome (Heydebrand 1980). Among points to be considered will be the role of the individual, the struggle between professional power and bureaucratic power (or managerial power), and the impact of a changing discourse on medicine, science and society. Perhaps most important is the need to locate a discussion of the parts within the context of the whole and, in so doing, recognize the importance of totality – the all-round domination of the whole over the parts (Lukács 1971).

Sociologists have often been concerned to identify the relationships of social structure and individual action. They have studied roles and personality, structural relationships and effective functions (Philips 1965). For example, how important are actors' own accounts, or, of what importance is an assessment of motive on an individual's part (Marshall 1981)? Some ideas of motive, to choose this as an example, will be highly deterministic (Marxist and Durkheimian); some stress the social structural aspect of the offering and interpreting of accounts (interactionalists) and some believe that actors' own accounts are all we can ever really know about the social world (ethnomethodologists) (Wallis and Bruce 1983). The picture grows more complicated if we add the distinction between action and intention. In other words, we may obtain an actor's own account that differs both from the real intention and from the objective result.

There have been numerous attempts to seek a methodological reconciliation of many of these different viewpoints; for example, Wallis and Bruce (1983) offered the following thesis:

> Explaining social action . . . entails understanding individual motiva-
> tion and belief, and thus taking actors' meanings, and what they say
> about them, seriously. Doing that, however, requires constant
> reference to a social and historical context. No one will adequately
> explain social action who does not understand how individuals
> interpret their world. But no one will understand how individuals
> interpret their world who is not aware of the social and historical
> context within which they do it.

An example of the sorts of problem encountered when these methodological complexities are related to specific examples can be seen if we seek to understand the apparent paradox of the Thatcher government in relation to the state. Thatcherism argues for a withdrawal of the state but practices the most interventionist state policy at least since the Second World War. David Marquand has argued that this is because of the primacy, even vis-à-vis the economic, of the cultural project of Thatcherism. Such a project requires an interventionist central government and is manifest in its aggressive stance towards local government and towards trade unions (*The Road from 1945*, BBC Radio 4, 1 April 1988). It is evident in its defence posture and in its elevation of 'policing for order' (Small 1987).

Sir John Hoskins, a long time adviser to Margaret Thatcher, argues that such contradictions are evident even within economic policy because the Thatcher project is a long-term one. In its early and middle phases reconstructing the economy does indeed need a measure of interventionism in, at least, creating and maintaining the necessary and sufficient conditions for economic change. For example, he would argue, the state needs to act to limit the capacity of trade unions to distort the labour market. It cannot rely entirely on the inhibiting impact of high levels of unemployment (*The Road from 1945*, BBC Radio 4, 1 April 1988).

But the dilemma for the Thatcherite project is that the economic dynamic it seeks has implication for the welfare state, and, of key importance in this analysis, for the NHS. The cultural struggle to facilitate changes in this area has not yet been won. Put simply, Thatcherism requires the use of the carrot and the stick. It requires a removal of the safety net. It wants, and needs, to challenge both Keynes and Beveridge. But if it is to succeed a general allegiance to the NHS, at least, needs to be changed. This becomes problematical because cultural allegiances may have autonomous status – they cannot be collapsed into the economic.

I am reminded of a philosopher of history, R.G. Collingwood (1924, p. 236), warning that contemporary history is unwritable because we know so much about it:

Contemporary history embarrasses a writer not only because he knows too much, but also because what he knows is too undigested, too unconnected, too atomic. It is only after close and prolonged reflection that we begin to see what was essential and what was important, to see why things happened as they did, and to write history instead of newspapers.

Collingwood's reservations, if followed, would eliminate most recent writing on social policy and certainly on the NHS. There are very good histories (Allsop 1984; Thane 1982), very good work on organization and policy (Ham 1985; Hunter 1980), considered treatments of the politics of health (Doyal and Pennell 1979; Iliffe 1983) and fascinating sociological analyses of medicine (Turner 1987). But things change so fast and much has to be written 'from the newspapers'.

Or, at least, it appears that things change so fast. One analysis of the NHS is that it is characterized by a considerable continuity. This is a possibility I address in my review of the public presentation of health policy in the 1980s, in my discussion about incrementalism and planning, and it is a subject I consider in my conclusion where I concentrate on the Department of Health (1989) White Paper, *Working for Patients*.

In preparing this work I have been much influenced by the wide range of literature available. I have taught about the NHS on Bradford University's MA in Social and Community Work Studies and Bradford's part-time BA in Social Sciences, and have been much informed by the contributions of students. I have used library facilities at Bradford and Leeds Universities, at the offices of Bradford District Health Authority, at Bradford Resource Centre, and at the DHSS in London. I have had many discussions, listened to many people talk and read a great deal of literature produced by groups campaigning against cuts in the NHS. The Strategy for Health Group provided the forum for many of these meetings. I have sought to acknowledge this range of influences in the text but much is hard to attribute in such a formal way. Members and officers of Bradford District Health Authority and other Bradfordians concerned with the provision of health care in their district spoke to me about the organization and practice of health care in one geographical area. All these influences have helped shape a book, the idiosyncrasies of which remain mine.

In my private life it is Isobel Conlon who has shared our home with the intrusive interloper a book becomes. Her help and support have been unfailing.

| PART I | Central Government and the National Health Service |

1 The Executive

Since its inception the National Health Service has been organized hierarchically. It is headed by a Minister of Health who, in 1988, assumed control from the then Secretary of State for Social Services. The Minister is assisted by junior ministers, and is supported by the staff of the Department of Health. Formally the Minister is responsible to Parliament, and the Social Services Select Committee of the House of Commons investigates various aspects of the Department's work.

If this is the barest structure it must be supplemented by the links with other ministries and departments of state via the Cabinet. The present Minister of Health is in the Cabinet. Prior to 1988 the NHS fell within the remit of the Department of Health and Social Security (DHSS), and its Secretary of State had always been in the Cabinet. There are bilateral contacts with ministries and with the Treasury and also contacts via the 'Star Chamber' system, where the claims of spending ministries and responses of the Treasury are discussed. There are also contacts via the organization of the governing party which acts both as a channel of communication and as a group seeking to maintain a sense of collective interest.

Moving further from the formal, the Minister is advised by various expert bodies and is also the focus (along with his department) of the concerted attentions of the pressure groups active in health. Finally, all this activity occurs within a particular political and ideological environment that will condition the options perceived to be possible in terms of policy-making and implementation within the NHS.

The executive may present as a straightforward organizational structure but in practice it is divided, in many cases fundamentally, by differences of approach, of vision and of interest. A considerable amount of the literature of political science concerns itself with the struggle between politician and bureaucrat. (I will try and resist quoting *Yes, Minister* too often!) There are divisions between the executive and the legislature and between public interest and pressure-group interests. The resulting conflicts are played out in this part of the organizational system as well as in the public realm of the media.

Within the executive there are evident different paradigms of change. One useful distinction is between an orientation which involves the identification and implementation of future goals, a planned and proactive stance towards change, called 'teleology' by one writer, and an assumption about change that involves the inevitable future and a need to make preparatory adaptation to it, called 'teleonomy' (Moore 1970). Both of these paradigms operate within a dominant metaphor of change (Nisbet 1969) which, for the duration of the NHS, has been one of 'growth' and 'progress'. If policies are proposed that are at odds with the dominant they have to be presented in such a way that they appear not to be. For example, policies of retrenchment, or of cuts, are portrayed either as temporary expedients which will be reversed when the inevitable improvement in the general economic climate occurs or as improvements that just look to the narrowly self-interested eye as cuts. One result of this is the development of a fascinating language of policy-making and presentation. We witness the arrival of terms like 'efficiency saving' and encounter a spirited debate about what a cut, as opposed to a rationalization of service, is.

For my immediate argument the importance of these linguistic constructions must be considered. Are they manifestations of a change in the dominant form of discourse in society? Are the New Right and Thatcherism seeking to establish a new social dynamic within which policy is formed? For example, is there a shift from ethical constructs forged under an alliance of paternalism and professionalism to ones generated by entrepreneurship and managerialism? Is there a new concern with the presentation of policy as opposed to its content, or even an emphasis on the language of policy-making as something located in expediency rather than justice?

There is an interesting literature present in the biographies and reminiscences of former ministers of health and secretaries of state. At first glance they appear a disparate lot. They include, for example, Aneurin Bevan (Minister of Health, 1945–51), Enoch Powell (1960–3), Richard Crossman (the first Secretary of State, 1968–70) and Barbara Castle (1974–6) (see Bevan 1952; Roth 1970; Crossman 1977; Castle 1976). But, despite the great differences in individual philosophy, the problems to be faced presented them with a considerably shared agenda. That is not to say that there was no scope for initiative. When not much can be done, in the short term, to change things fundamentally then some of the smaller changes in style – or in priorities – can seem very important to workers in the NHS, to the public and to political commentators.

I want to begin this look at the executive with some comments on Norman Fowler, who was appointed Secretary of State by Mrs Thatcher in

1981 – succeeding Patrick Jenkin, who had held office from the 1979 election. It is more difficult to assess the contribution of a current, or very recent, Secretary of State than of one from the past because of the absence of those considered diaries and memoirs that prove so useful from other people (Crossman and Castle, for example). Norman Fowler is also difficult because he was not an ideologue in the sense of having committed his ideas on the welfare state to detailed presentation, unlike Bevan and Powell. Without the aid of these routes to understanding, it is difficult to get a sense, except through deductive reasoning, of such areas as the debates in Cabinet, the relationship with other departments of state and the contact between the Secretary of State and his advisers in the DHSS. It is also difficult to identify any underlying philosophy or guide to action.

An example of the complexity of contemporary policy analysis might be provided by seeking an assessment of the changing role of the Treasury in influencing DHSS policy. During the Thatcher governments there has been an apparent increase in the power of the Treasury over the spending ministries. The Treasury has become more directly interventionist, aided by its increasing employment of economists. It may be that this changed relationship between departments is a reflection of the particular personalities of their respective heads, it may be the result of a prevalent balance of power within the Cabinet, or it may be a manifestation of a fundamental change of orientation within the whole administration and so be of key importance in evaluating likely developments in planning and policy-making (Hearn and Small 1984).

There is a characteristic dilemma for heads of spending departments in that they will owe their advancement to the ruling party and its leader but will gain their status from an ability to support their own department against the encroachments and opposition of others. If the overall avowed philosophy of the government is one which aims to limit expenditure and to redefine the role of the welfare state in society then that problem is compounded. Fowler has to become a monetarist who wants to spend money. He becomes someone who is always making 'special case' pleas. His dilemma is that he finds himself in the Cabinet where all the spending departments are doing the same!

Cabinet politics never appears more ingenuous, more like a game, than during the annual spending round when this 'wheeler-dealing' goes on. Resolution is sought in two ways. The first is the special-case pleading mentioned above. The second is the use of a particular form of language or a manipulation of figures to indicate that either things are not as bad as they appear or they are not as bad as they might have been. The term 'efficiency savings' is just one of many used. Cuts in funding, it implies, will be at the expense of waste and patient care will not suffer.

There has been an endless struggle over figures on expenditure. The government presents increased expenditure figures, while critics say that these are misleading, based on inappropriate data, or are too selective. If the politics of presentation is of key importance, and the way information is communicated is indicative of fundamentals in terms of the working of the executive, it is worth looking in more detail at how Norman Fowler and the DHSS have specifically used figures.

Control of information is one of the key organizational functions of the executive. It is certainly something that can be used to define the parameters of debate. In health – and in many other areas of social policy, most notably employment – the government's presentation of figures in specific ways has left its opponents struggling. The result has been a sterile debate in which the initiative remains firmly with the government. It issues figures saying that it is spending more than ever before on the NHS, the Opposition says that it is not – or at least not really – and the politics of health is subsumed in an incomprehensible struggle over semantics.

Until 1978 full figures were published annually in the *Health and Personal Social Services Statistics for England*. This has stopped – only one volume has emerged since then, in 1982, and this referred to figures relevant to 1980. The result is that, although other figures are still made available by the DHSS, they are not as detailed and do not have the same continuity of presentation, and hence facility for comparison, as they did before.

An example is provided by the leaflet *The Health Service in England* issued by the DHSS (1984a) via regional health authority chairmen and designed to reassure that the NHS was 'developing and improving'. This document presented figures from two years only, 1983 (the most recent year the document could draw on) and 1978 (the year before the Conservatives returned to power). There are many problems in making use of the figures presented. Things take a considerable time to change in the NHS. In understanding health we must take into account more than the episodic treatment of ill health. Apparent improvements may be due to factors other than those within the control of the NHS. So when the figures point to significant reductions in perinatal mortality rates between 1978 and 1983 (a fall of 33 per cent) it is important to put this into the context of a much longer gradual reduction and a rapid rate of reduction from 1976 not 1978.

As numbers reduce it is more likely that dramatic statistical changes will be demonstrated (if 5000 people in one year die of a particular condition and the next year 4500, then 500 lives is only a 10 per cent reduction; if ten years later only 1000 people a year die and this reduces to 800 then 200 lives is presented as 20 per cent).

In July 1986, in response to criticism in the House of Commons, the Prime Minister cited low infant mortality rates as indicative of the healthy state of the NHS (*Guardian*, 7 July 1986). It was a claim much disputed by professionals and by pressure groups. Doctors argued that an advance in medical knowledge had led to a general reduction in perinatal mortality in much of the world. The United Kingdom's position would place it in the middle of a league table of industrialized countries. But in other related areas the UK had not done as well. Other countries had seen a reduction in the number of babies of low birth-weight but in the UK the figure had remained at approximately 7 per cent since the mid-1960s (in Scandinavia the figure is 4 per cent). Babies born of unskilled workers are twice as likely to die as babies born into the professional classes, and the gap is wider than it was 15 years ago. In 1984, 7500 babies were stillborn or died during the first weeks of life. If the risk of death for all babies was the same as it is for those born into social class 1 then about 3000 babies lives would be saved each year. There is an acute shortage of doctors and nurses and a shortage of equipment.

The Maternity Alliance, an umbrella lobbying organization for all the pressure groups concerned with childbirth and infant welfare, estimates that there is a shortfall of 40 per cent in the number of intensive care baby cots in the UK. In many hospitals 75 per cent of specialized equipment has been provided by charity. One consultant at King's College Hospital, London, said that 'he now spent a large part of his time attending charity fundraising events instead of caring for sick children' (*Guardian*, 7 July 1986).

NHS figures are quoted as numbers and not as rates, not as proportions of people who need services. If service offered is not related to an assessment of need then there is no way of identifying the extent of unmet need. It is generally accepted that some basic demographic changes will of themselves increase need. The increase in the number of elderly in the population is one such change. Although disputed in some quarters, there are strongly supported arguments that some economic changes, particularly the rise in unemployment, also increase need. Figures are chosen selectively. For example, increases in the number of patients accepted for kidney treatment are not presented alongside the figures on the extent to which this treatment was successful, nor with figures on how many remain to be treated. DHSS (1984a) referred to increases in the number of coronary bypass operations and the establishment of three new spinal injuries centres, but glossed over less glamorous or innovative operations.

It has always been the case that some areas of medical endeavour are more popular with practitioners than others. This was evident in the early Voluntary Hospitals (Widgery 1979). Many of these areas also assume a glamour and attract a measure of popular interest and support that may protect them from some of the vicissitudes of changing economic fortune. Status has been one of the factors presented in defence of units threatened with cuts within the NHS. It is a fine line to tread – status and popularity may also mean that a facility could attract voluntary or charitable support. Both Stoke Mandeville (spinal injuries) and Tadworth (heart surgery) hospitals have been threatened with cuts since 1979.

Fundamentally the issue is that finance for the NHS is determined by economic decisions and not by an assessment of real health need. There will thus always be rationing and allocation decisions to make. If high-status facilities are reprieved it is not with an overall provision of extra money (or at least not usually) but at the expense of less visible services and facilities, which are deprived of the funds they need.

It is hard to identify a determining construct to help make planning decisions about the allocation of scarce resources. There are long-term policy aims, the shift of resources via the Resource Allocation Working Party (RAWP), a prioritization of the mental illness and mental handicap services, the development of community care. But there are also areas identified as in urgent need, perhaps because they are seen to be politically expedient.

There are also the ongoing pressures of cost increases that are above the average. In the period between 1965 and 1975, according to Ian Gough (1979, pp. 84–94), there was an apparent increase in spending on the NHS of 314 per cent. Of that, 244 per cent was due to general inflation. The rest was made up of a combination of four factors. The first factor was rising relative costs. Costs in the welfare state as a whole have tended to rise at a rate higher than that of general inflation. The second was population changes, specifically the changing age structure of the population. Briefly, there are more elderly people in the community and they require, on average, a greater share of health care resources. The third was the spending demands of new and improved services. Hospitals that acquired body scanners, often as gifts from charitable efforts, for example, were always wary of the revenue cost implications of running them. They now find that as the body scanners wear out they do not have a charity waiting to replace them but have to meet what is now an expectation within their district for such a service. The fourth was pressure from growing social needs, both the social costs of economic change – from industrial pollution to thalidomide – and the costs of recession, most notably in increased unemployment. The end result is that Gough identifies a real increase in expenditure of 27 per cent over a ten-year period.

The NHS as an organization has not worked out a means of acknowledging the problem of a finance-led planning system in an environment of increasing financial cost. I will look in a subsequent chapter at the attempts it has made, and is making, but will suggest that the majority of its efforts seem to be rhetorical rather than actual.

There are many areas of adjustment to figures that make comparisons with previous figures difficult. DHSS (1984a) quotes a 12 per cent increase in in-patient cases between 1978 and 1983. But what is an in-patient case? It is not a record of the number of persons treated in a year but is the figure arrived at by deducting the number of deaths in hospital from the number of admissions. This means that if the same person is treated several times in a year that person is counted once on each admission. A 12 per cent increase may therefore simply be arrived at by discharging people before they are ready and then having to readmit them later in the year.

The same sort of complications exist in looking at staff figures. The DHSS in 1984 reported a 13 per cent increase in numbers of nursing and midwifery staff (measured in whole-time equivalents). But during this time the length of the working week was reduced, so inevitably if you measure staff by number of hours worked it looks as if more staff have been employed (Radical Statistics Health Group (RSHG) 1985; see also RSHG 1980; 1987).

If the control of information and the presentation of figures is of key importance in understanding the role of the executive, the second main area of executive concern is that of living with, and seeking an operational policy through, the many and often conflicting demands made upon it. In order better to illustrate some of these issues I will look at those areas that appeared to concern Secretary of State Norman Fowler in a four-month period in the summer of 1983. It is a period I have chosen at random and, in any longer-term analysis, would not necessarily appear crucial.

In the spring of 1983 the Secretary of State had been speaking expansively about a period of financial stringency being over. A spending freeze was about to be reversed so that more money could be spent on services for patients. He was encouraging health administrators to prepare buildings because funds would be available for them to be used in the near future. Such encouragement included advice to catch up on repairs and redecoration and followed adverse criticism on the existence of empty wards because of shortages of staff in areas where there was a clear demand for services (*Guardian*, 8 July 1983). But this mood was short-lived as pressure was exerted from the Treasury for another round of cuts. In this atmosphere the DHSS appeared particularly vulnerable. It had been embarrassed by an overspending on that part of its budget allocated to the Family Practitioner Service. This section of the budget was not cash-limited and so was difficult for the DHSS to control.

The result of the discussions in Cabinet, and between the DHSS and the Treasury, was that there was to be a cut of £97 million in the NHS budget. This was to be found by a reduction in revenue costs, cutting back staff and spending on goods and services, and a reduction in the capital costs of the proposed hospital building programme. Given the conflicts described above, it will not be surprising to find that, in announcing these reductions, Fowler was to point out that they would not damage patient care (*Sunday Times*, 10 July 1983). Once more the attempt to reconcile the inevitable with the unacceptable – cuts with the reluctance to admit to cuts – produced claims from the Secretary of State that the main effect would be on administrative, clerical, maintenance and other support staff as well as on the amounts spent on supplies and energy. He claimed that the required cuts could be obtained without any more ward or hospital closures or a lengthening of hospital waiting lists. Jobs would be lost but he did not as yet know how many. Health authorities and certainly the health trade unions did not seem to share the assessment of the 'limited impact' of these cuts (*Guardian*, 12 July 1983).

The dilemma for the NHS in a situation like this is that the possibility of making and implementing long-term plans is severely limited. One can make plans that are conditional on a certain level of financing but that level has to be predictable over time. In this case the health authorities were committed to an increase in the number of consultants employed within the NHS, particularly in certain disciplines and in certain areas. Employing consultants carries with it other revenue costs and can often lead, within a specific hospital, or indeed a district, to the development of a specialism that can have both revenue and capital cost implications. Consultants are appointed by the regional health authority and enjoy a measure of autonomy *vis-à-vis* the district in which they work. So the dilemma, in a time of cuts, was that the scope for planning staff reductions was considerably limited by this prior commitment. If there were to be staff reductions at the same time as health authorities had to employ more consultants then savings would have to be made by reducing numbers of other lower-paid grades (more people for the same saving). Further, a cut in the hospital building programme would mean a concentration on sites already in use which would run contrary to a longer-term policy aim of seeking decentralized community care.

It would appear that one of the major roles of the executive is to introduce short-term considerations into a previously determined long-term policy, and in such a way as often to jeopardize the latter. It is such a role that often prompts NHS planners and administrators to speak wistfully of the ideal of 'taking the politics out of health'. In this particular case the DHSS, having appeared to lose the initiative to the Treasury because of problems in managing its own expenditure, did respond with a proposal that it thought would avoid some of the problems of unpredictable revenue costs in the future. It suggested the establishment of manpower targets, a new departure, though consistent with the already established practice of operating to cash limits and expenditure targets based on resources rather than need. In these circumstances it was envisaged that a cut of 0.5 per cent in front-line staff (doctors, nurses and paramedics) and a cut of 0.75 per cent in ancillary staff (porters, kitchen staff, laundry staff and gardeners) would meet the Treasury requirements. But, given the position concerning consultants described above and the longer-term policy of encouraging certain areas of specialism, it did look – and the media were quick to point this out – that these cuts would mean that 'Doctors were next for the NHS axe' (*Guardian*, 23 July 1983).

If the debate so far had been primarily located in the private realm of DHSS–Treasury discussion it now shifted into the public sphere, motivated by those opposed to the cuts. At times this sort of shift can help the spending ministry fend off the Treasury and indeed might be set in process by judicious 'leaks' from the department concerned. The potential to exploit public pressure appeared greater in health than in many other areas of government policy. The Conservatives wished both to cut and to be seen as protecting the NHS.

This appeared to be the dominant position in the Cabinet and certainly one that Norman Fowler was identified with. He had made it known that he thought the NHS 'a good thing' and had argued upon taking office against a major transformation of its financing. He was an avowed admirer of Enoch Powell's *A New Look at Medicine and Politics* (Powell 1966). Powell combined an appreciation of *Realpolitik* with a theoretical and ethical appreciation of something he defined as public duty. Powell had also believed that a health minister would have little chance of success in a dispute with a chancellor. But if this is the case it has not stopped each successive health minister seeking to fight the Department's corner.

At the time the cuts were being considered Parliament was in recess and the usual briefing system for Westminster-based journalists in abeyance. Consequently there appeared considerable opportunity for opponents of the government's policy to take the initiative. One government critic from the Labour Party (Opposition members starved of media space know that if they forgo their summer in Tuscany they will have journalists queuing up to report their every word) described the government proposals as akin to practising on the NHS 'a desperate form of mediaeval medicine . . . where you bleed the patient to save his life'. Rodney Bickerstaff, General Secretary of NUPE, broadened the debate by identifying the government's disregard for the NHS with the observation that in the last resort 'they did not have to rely on it' (*Guardian*, 24 September 1983).

Opposition was also growing from a number of health authorities. They were worried that there was not the slack the government appeared to be assuming or hoping existed and that the cuts would inevitably lead to reductions in services to patients. Some authorities were also keen to exploit what they saw as contradictions in the policy. For example, the West Midlands Regional Health Authority believed that it could create another 2100 jobs while remaining within its cash limits. Cash limits and manpower limits might not coincide and the Authority was pushing the government to ask which took precedence (*Guardian*, 23 September 1983). The dilemma for the Secretary of State was that it appeared authorities might be able to reduce services rather than staff and if they did so this would not accord with the picture of 'no damage' the government was determined to portray.

The government was not keen to precipitate a major argument with the health authorities. It had less to fear from trouble with one isolated district, such as occurred when the Lambeth, Southwark and Lewisham District

Health Authority refused to comply with an earlier round of cuts and was suspended. But now the government saw the possibility of more widespread opposition centred on these complex issues.

An interesting difference in the use of language illustrates what was at the heart of the dispute. The government always spoke of seeking a 1 per cent reduction in NHS staffing. It appealed to a 'common-sense' belief that in an organization as large as the NHS it must be possible to make reductions as small as this by eliminating waste and tightening up efficiency. The health authorities spoke of it not as a 1 per cent cut but as the loss of 4837 jobs. Each of those job losses would involve discussions about who must go, what do they do and who would do it when they were gone. The trade unions and professional organizations appeared ready to question every job loss and, not surprisingly, the authorities found the prospect of entering into these negotiations daunting.

Another voice of opposition was the British Medical Association (BMA), which was particularly critical of the abandonment of long-term planning objectives. Short-term decisions may appear necessary and expedient but they would jeopardize the long-term effective running of the NHS. Specifically, the BMA objected to the imposition of 'arbitrary' cash cuts in the middle of a budgetary year. One result of such cuts, it said, was to necessitate the shift of money from capital accounts to minimize the short-term damage to services. But to shift capital funds was to put at risk long-decided programmes of rebuilding, re-equipping and restructuring. The example the BMA presented to support this argument, one clearly related to its professional interests, was that there would be a reduction in teaching posts and beds in teaching hospitals as part of efforts to save cash. That would be detrimental to the long-term provision of enough specialists, in enough disciplines, to maintain the required service in the future (*Guardian*, 21 October 1983).

I have suggested that during this period the Secretary of State had first to struggle with the Treasury and then with the Opposition, the trade unions, professional organizations and a considerable proportion of the health authorities. In the early stages the upper hand seemed to be with the Treasury and Fowler's response to the pressure put on him and to the contradictions inherent in his position was to adopt the rhetorical solution. He would make cuts but they would not hurt services. He did have the alternative of fighting in Cabinet, either alone in making a special-case plea, or in concert with other heads of spending ministries. He no doubt decided that the circumstances required his being a good Cabinet man. No doubt he was mindful of the last revolt by heads of spending departments in 1981. They lost and many were reshuffled just before a round of bilateral negotiations with the Treasury, thus seriously weakening the position of the spending ministries (*Guardian*, 25 July 1983).

Norman Fowler seemed to have learnt political lessons from 1981. His appointment to the Cabinet had been something of a surprise. He had supported Edward Heath in the leadership election that saw Mrs Thatcher victorious. Commentators at the time saw him as a lightweight, as 'an embodiment of the Peter Principle that decrees people naturally rise in an organisation to the level of incompetence (clots find their slots)' (*Sunday Times*, 19 February 1984).

He was also taking office at a time when a major change in the nature of Cabinet government was occurring, a change that one could assume would not be to the advantage of the spending ministries like the DHSS. Mrs Thatcher was constructing 'the most streamlined, personalised government since the Second World War' (*Observer*, 3 January 1988). Under Mrs Thatcher the Cabinet has met between 40 and 45 times a year, about half as often as in the governments that preceded hers. In its first six years 160 ministerial committees were set up (in the same period Attlee's government had seen 450 and Wilson's over 250). In 1984 the Cabinet Office prepared only 60 or 70 classified papers for senior ministers – one-sixth as many as in an average year in the 1950s. Between 1979 and the end of 1987 Mrs Thatcher had appointed 24 of Whitehall's 27 permanent secretaries. She knew all the key officials and could, if she wished, bypass the Minister and talk to them directly (*Observer*, 3 January 1988).

This strong centralizing dynamic, evident within the executive, is manifest in both the organizational changes that have been an important feature of Thatcherism and in the maintenance of an ideological agenda concerned to reconstruct the atmosphere of policy-making at the centre. I would argue that this centralizing tendency is also evident in all parts of the NHS. Indeed, changes in the nature of Cabinet government can be presented as a paradigm for the attempted reconstruction of the state at all levels, including, for example, the introduction of general management into the NHS.

A centralization of decision-making and the development of the management function within the NHS closes off some of the traditional routes of seeking political influence. One of the most notable changes since 1979 has been the way pressure groups in health, the doctors for example, have had to shift from an increasingly inaccessible private route into the public sphere in order to influence policy. The public discourse on health policy has been increasingly strident as, in particular, the professions see an emerging influence in policy-making to counter the central role they have occupied in the past. They have pursued two strategies: an attempt to co-opt management as an adjunct to professional power; and a heightened public profile from which they can voice opposition to those policies deemed against their professional interest.

The possibilities of using public debate provided Norman Fowler with both problems and opportunities. As the discussion of health policy emerged from the Cabinet, from bilateral discussions with the Treasury and from the 'Star Chamber', there was a period in which the Secretary of State was very much in the public eye and could use this position to strengthen his hand in the remaining detail of negotiations within the executive. He could present further cuts as being politically damaging and remind his colleagues that the Conservative Party as a whole seemed to have decided that the NHS should be seen to be 'safe in their hands'. This might involve an appeal over the heads of the Cabinet to the Conservative Party in Parliament. This is a risky move that is best pursued by hint and suggestion because it may excite the combined opposition of the rest of the Cabinet and of back-benchers in favour of a more rigid implementation of the agreed economic policy.

Most criticism of the Secretary of State from his Conservative Party colleagues during this period was directed at his management of the cuts, which they feared had united the usually moderate nurses and doctors with the more usually militant ancillary workers (*Guardian*, 8 October 1983). It appears in such matters to be axiomatic that if you can divide and rule you should. Consequently these criticisms were ones Fowler could not take lightly – they addressed his central skills as a politician. Indeed he was quick to respond using the simple and well-tried expedient of announcing that he would introduce a different approach to planning next time and that the job losses would be concentrated in the ancillary grades (*Guardian*, 13 October 1983).

The period described above is not an unusual one, it is not one that would only exist with Norman Fowler as Secretary of State or under a Conservative government. There have been many similar struggles between the Department of State and the Treasury. Richard Crossman and Roy Jenkins were the leading protagonists in a well-documented earlier struggle (Crossman 1977). What differs is style and not content. For example, all secretaries of state seek a way out of the complexities of effecting change in the NHS by proposing some sort of reorganization, be it structural or administrative, and all struggle with the problems of a limited budget and the inflexibility of long-term financial commitments. The NHS has always been essentially political in that it is very much in the public eye and the public perception of its state of well-being has an impact on the popularity of the political party in power. Such a high profile creates problems but also opportunities for the minister in charge.

The NHS, perhaps more than any other institution in contemporary society, is perceived ideologically/symbolically, and not scrutinized for effectiveness save by those people who need its services. Even then criticism of specifics rarely translates to the general. Patients may complain about the length of waiting lists or the infantilizing and discourteous treatment they receive in hospitals but they do not link that with any fundamental criticism of the NHS as a whole. Perhaps they think that is all they deserve or that their experience is an unfortunate, isolated, occurrence. (Most letters of complaint received by chairmen of district health authorities relate to these two complaints. The normal response is that pressure of work accounts for the discourtesy and a shortage of funds, not within the control of the district, for the waiting lists. A collective problem or a problem with the possibility of solution is not recognized.)

The resolution of the evident disputes between the Treasury and the DHSS in 1983 appeared to be a victory for the Treasury, but only just. The government was able to maintain the stance of cuts being of peripheral importance and Norman Fowler was able to maintain that his department had come through the period virtually unscathed.

Apart from this area of concern, the Secretary of State and his Health Minister – Norman Fowler had persuaded Mrs Thatcher to appoint Kenneth Clarke to this post – were involved in 1983 and 1984 in a number of other controversies. They were seeking to emphasize cost effectiveness in the NHS. This led to moves to force competitive tendering for hospital laundry and for cleaning services but it also produced an attack on drug company profits of an order that had not been mounted since Enoch Powell was minister (*New Statesman*, 1 June 1984, p. 15). This was not symptomatic of a general attack on big business in health, indeed the Secretary of State was very generous to British Oxygen in his enhancing of its monopoly position as supplier of medical gases. During this same period Clarke and Fowler did appear to act energetically in responding to criticisms of the quality of doctors' night-time deputizing services. By February 1984 Norman Fowler was even ready to disagree with the publicly expressed position of the Prime Minister that girls of under 16 should not be prescribed the contraceptive pill.

Formally the NHS is a centralized organization. The executive is responsible for making policy, for resource allocation and for the scrutiny of performance. It controls finance and appoints key personnel. But the executive itself cannot simply be considered as a monolith. It operates within a political arena one of whose features is the number of different, often conflicting, imperatives ostensibly adhered to by the government. Further, there is some attempt to devolve decision-making and responsibility. The extent of this varies according to the perceived political sensitivity of issues and to the intensity of the centralizing and interventionist tendencies of the government of the day.

The very first NHS circular sent from the Ministry of Health to regional hospital boards (Health Circular RHB(47)1) referred to the latter as being the minister's agents but hoped they would 'feel from the outset . . . a lively sense of independent responsibility'. Regional hospital boards were expected to allow hospital management committees a maximum autonomy in regard to day-to-day administration, with boards reserving the wider policy decisions. But such a system has consistently presented problems and uncertainties. To be allowed autonomy when the DHSS thinks it appropriate and only in areas it chooses not to concern itself with is a precarious autonomy.

Some elements evident in the process within the executive, and in relations between the centre and the units of the NHS, accord with a 'popular' belief that in state bureaucracies there must be waste. Such a stance not only seeks to ally itself with an aspect of what has been called 'authoritarian popularism' (Hall and Jacques 1983) but also seeks sanction from the academic Right. Indeed Niskanen (1973), one of the New Right's major economists and an adviser to President Reagan, seems to make the categories synonymous. For him bureaucracy is a phenomenon that generates its own needs, over and above the purpose for which it ostensibly exists. Consequently there always exists unnecessary capacity and improvement can be made simply by cutting. He offers a rationalization for less government irrespective of the need for a lengthy study of agency function.

It can also be argued that the nature of changing policy in health is understandable as part of another process evident within the Right. This is the long-term strategy designed to introduce the private sector into more and more areas of health care in the pursuit of profit and under the banner of the encouragement of choice. Certainly this is in accord with the work developed in the Institute of Economic Affairs in the 1960s and 1970s. It is generally considered the preserve of conspiracy theorists to equate cuts in the NHS with a deliberate attempt to make private health care seem more attractive. Conspiracy theories are rather frowned on by the Left at the moment. They are replaced by theories that explore the roots of the Right in popular consciousness (Campbell 1987). But the deliberations of the 1982 Conservative Think Tank, made public by means of a number of leaks, go some way towards making such theories respectable again.

This was a group looking at various aspects of 'family policy and the future of the welfare state'. A leaked draft circular spoke of hiving off parts of the NHS, including geriatric care (*Guardian*, 17 February 1983). It seemed clear that, at the very least, the purpose of this leak was to test the popular reaction and to sound out the enthusiasm of the private sector for taking on such a role. The result was negative and this excited the fear of electoral retribution. It seemed to persuade the government that if it wished to pursue such a policy it would have to do it more slowly, having built more of a constituency for such changes. This is an example of that clash of conspiracy theory and authoritarian popularism and the clash between a political agenda that is dominated by a wish to restructure the British state and attitudes towards welfare in particular and a more long-standing political programme of electoral success and calculated expediency.

2 The Central Administration and the National Health Service

If the role of the Minister/Secretary of State shows both continuity and change this is also the case for the central administration, now in the Department of Health, having in 1988 been separated from Social Security.

Any consideration of the nature of bureaucracy needs to acknowledge Max Weber (1948; 1949) and it is with his model that I will begin. Bureaucracy, he argued, developed from, and replaced, an earlier social form based on personal subjugation, nepotism, cruelty and a capricious use of subjective judgements. It was the best administrative form for the rational and effective pursuit of organizational goals. He identified a number of discrete elements that were tied together in an overarching phenomenon of rationality. That rationality embraced two slightly different things. First, the rationality of bureaucracy was that it maximized technical efficiency. The rules defined the most appropriate means to realize organizational ends, they were based on up-to-date technical knowledge and directed the behaviour of members along the most efficient lines. Second, bureaucracy was a system of social control, or authority, that was acceptable to members because they saw the rules as rational, fair and impartial – a legal rational value system (Albrow 1970).

Since Weber's presentation of his bureaucratic ideal type, both his work and bureaucracy itself have been much examined and criticized. One criticism has been that many bureaucratic organizations have been found to work inefficiently. R.K. Merton (1957) demonstrated that the structure of bureaucratic organizations becomes inflexible because members adhere to the rules in a ritualistic manner and they elevate these above the goals they are designed to realize. Specialization often fosters a narrow outlook which cannot solve new problems, colleagues within departments develop feelings of loyalty to each other and their departments and promote these group interests when they can. Crozier (1964) develops this argument to show that bureaucracies embody vicious circles of decreasing efficiency and effectiveness. His argument is that within bureaucracies groups of colleagues attempt to maximize their own freedom of action by paying lip-service to the rules but ignoring the spirit behind them and bending them when they can. They can withhold or distort information so that senior managers do not know what is going on. They, in turn, create more rules to regulate what is beneath them and about which they have suspicions. Such rules are made in an 'arbitrary or personal manner' and are legitimized as being directed against those they suspect of failing to promote organizational goals. The result is that the organization becomes more and more rigid but may still fail to control subordinates.

W.G. Bennis (1966) developed some of these criticisms, making four points of particular relevance to bureaucracy. The model allows no problem in the integration of individual needs into management goals. It presents the individual as a passive instrument to be disregarded. The bureaucratic model does not sufficiently allow for the complexities of power relations; in its emphasis on legal rational power it underestimates the importance of an implicit use of coercive power. It replaces what is a confusing, ambiguous, complex web of coercion, legal codes and differing competencies into a too straightforward hierarchy. According to the model bureaucracies operate the rule of hierarchy to resolve conflicts between horizontal groups. They surround all this with appeals to loyalty to the organization. This may work when the environment is stable, although it remains too simple a model even then, but it allows for only a haphazard response to change.

It is a model that misses out both the context within which the bureacracy works and the informal life, the life of the organization outside the formal structural relationships. Two observations will illustrate. The first relates to the lack of meaningful party political debate about the NHS that has characterised so much of its history. Writing in general terms about the relationship of a democratic politics and bureaucracy, Rosa Luxemburg has pointed to the absence of the free struggle of opinion resulting in public life falling asleep and the bureaucracy remaining as the only active element (Frolich 1983, p. 249). If such characteristics could be attributed to the NHS then this would explain the considerable power exercised by the bureaucracy. On the relationship of the formal and informal life of organizations, the American journalist, Izzy Stone, advised those encountering public officials to listen to what they say informally, to take more notice of the things they say officially and in public (because these are things over which they can be called to question) but, above all, to study what they do (Lloyd 1986, p. 19).

Before looking specifically at the DHSS as it operated in the recent past, I want to look a little more at the analysis of bureaucracy presented by Niskanen and introduced in Chapter 1. This will help link this chapter with the presentation of the ideas of the New Right as they relate to health and welfare.

Niskanen presents a picture of the utility-maximizing individual. Producers and consumers are usually categorized in this way – as essentially self-interested and seeking to maximize their utilities. This translates to bureaucracies in the figure of the 'budget-maximizing bureaucrat' (he is largely talking about senior officials and primarily about the United States). These utilities include salary and other advantages of holding office including patronage and public reputation, but all can be expressed more simply because they are encompassed in the overriding concern to maximize the size of the department's budget. A bigger budget means all utilities are more satisfied. This inflation of the budget will occur irrespective of the real cost of supplying the department output and, in effect, there will be evident a bureaucratic profit which can be used to further other goals such as patronage, power and status.

The possibility for the development of this phenomenon arises because the relationship between bureaucrat and legislator is one of a bilateral monopoly, the sole supplier and the sole buyer. The advantages in this relationship lie with the supplier, the bureaucracy, because they have a monopoly not only over output but also over information about the true cost of supply. They build into their departmental estimates a measure of profit and hence the size of the budget becomes larger than is socially optimal (Thrasher 1984). The immediate implications of this analysis are that cuts can always be made without of necessity harming services, and that privatization would break down the sole-supplier situation that allows this bureaucratic profit to be established.

Niskanen's presentation of a budget-maximizing bureaucrat has been criticized on a number of grounds. Perhaps bureaucrats have 'life time aspirations' which may stifle short-term budgetary expansionism (Margolis 1975). Perhaps they identify more with particular policies than with the size of budgets. Margolis (1975), again, talks of 'mission-committed' bureaucrats and Goodin (1982) argues that policies and not budgets are a better basis for understanding the relationship between politicians and bureaucrats. Perhaps they identify the changing social dynamic and recognize that status can be gained by acting in accord with the government policy objectives of a reduction in the size of a particular service. They may gain status from being an efficient propagator and manager of cutbacks.

Another criticism of Niskanen may be to suggest that the legislature is more active than his model permits. This may not necessarily be the legislature as a whole but may be a committee of it. It is indeed the case, as we shall see when examining the legislature, that the committee system does allow for a closer scrutiny than the Niskanen model would presume. Conversely, it may be that the close relationship between a committee and a department produce an alliance in which the committee feels its needs furthered by the continued growth and success of the department. Its prime allegiance is to the department and not to the legislature as a whole who it may feel to be ill informed on this important subject area.

There are two ways I wish to pursue Niskanen's argument. The first is to look at the distribution of power and the nature of decision-making within the DHSS. It may be that the decisions the bureaucracy proposes are not made by one individual but are an aggregate that may reflect no one person's utility needs even if each individual was pursuing them. Perhaps a bureaucracy is not as straightforwardly hierarchical as the model suggests. For example, if budget increases do benefit the bureaucracy head they may mean more work for lower-level officials without an increase in their individual utility to offset this. Further, it may be that individual officials have an investment in a part of the budget only and may wish to see it increased even at the expense of another item within the overall department budget. If such practices exist this suggests a much more pluralist and conflict-ridden model of bureaucratic process and outcome.

A department as huge as the DHSS not only has the possibilities of such conflicts between personnel, but it is also divided fundamentally in terms of the functions it carries out. In two of its three main sections it can be categorized as a control agency, that is, in its relations with the personal social services (where this is mediated by the local authorities) and in the NHS (where the line of responsibility and accountability is directly with the department via appointed bodies at region and district). Its third branch is concerned with the administration of pensions and benefits and here it acts as a transfer agency. It would follow that budget maximization in the transfer agency is an unlikely aim even if it is pursued in relation to control-agency functions.

One area to examine is the possibility of identifying utility with the exercise of power, with the size of the sphere of influence, as opposed to a straightforward financial count of budget size. This would then have to be related to an atmosphere in which the dominant political orthodoxy is one of attempts to reduce the size of the public sector. That there have been problems in achieving such budget reduction may be because of a flaw in the New Right model and the contradictions inherent in state activity. It may be because of the dominance of incrementalism in the planning and decision-making process which prevents governments, at least in the short or medium term, reversing an upward trend in public expenditure. Or it may be, as Niskanen argues, that, irrespective of government policy, the agenda of the bureaucracy is to increase its budget.

The relationship between the centre and the periphery in the NHS has been a varied one. There have been times when the centre has wished to encourage more independence, for example in encouraging regions to act as more stratgic planning bodies after the introduction of the Hospital Plan in 1962 (Ministry of Health 1962). In that plan it was envisaged that the Ministry would issue guidance on the concept of the district general hospital and the bed norms to be used in planning such facilities. The Ministry would give advice on design and would have to give its permission for major schemes but within that the boards could choose where and when to build the hospitals. But central control was increased via the earmarking of money for specific long-stay services after the publication of reports into the condition of long-stay hospitals, most notably the report into allegations of ill treatment at Ely Hospital Cardiff (DHSS 1969).

In its control of finance the scope for the exercise of central power is limited by the restraints of incremental budgeting and by the problem of enforcing action on the part of the regions and districts. But earmarking is a powerful centralizing device and reflects the political reality that even if regions and districts are delegated planning powers it is unlikely that the DHSS and the politicians will resist the inclination to intervene to respond to issues of public concern and hence of political importance. DHSS (1969) not only produced earmarking of funds for that sector (earmarking had been done before) but also led to the Secretary of State's decision to establish the Hospital Advisory Service. This was set up in 1969 after battles with senior Civil Servants. This, and subsequent special committees that had been set up, were often perceived by those who established them and by the Civil Servants who opposed them, as devices for getting past the entrenched ways and narrow advice of permanent officials. One of those suggestions that produces most horror in the Civil Service is that, like in the USA, incoming ministers ought to be able to make some political appointments to top posts within their ministries (or at least to such posts as would secure them the advice they need on the operations within their department and the political implications of certain policy decisions).

Ministers have always looked outside the department for advice and indeed since the 1960s advisers have been appointed more formally, often to provide a source of alternative briefing. Harold Wilson identified six functions for advisers. They would act

> as a sieve, examining papers for politically sensitive or other important problems; as a deviller, chasing Ministers' requests or instructions; as a thinker on medium and long term planning; as a party contact man, keeping in touch especially with the parties' own research department; as a pressure group contact man; and as a speech writer (quoted in Blackstone 1979).

Apart from begging the question whether such a person would ever have any time off, this list is indicative of what the Civil Service does not do for the minister, or does in such a way that the minister is not sure of the objectivity of the advice given. It also identifies other possible sources of influence, of countervailing power to that of the bureaucracy: the ruling party, perhaps via its research department; pressure groups; other ministers; and public opinion.

One of the ongoing jokes in *Yes, Minister* is based on the accepted understanding that ministries are just there to act as conduits for pressure groups to get to the centre of power, or at least to the place where resources are allocated. The Ministry of Agriculture lobbies for the farmers, they say, the Ministry of Defence for the arms industry, and so on. As for the DHSS, that lobbies for the doctors (at least that branch of the DHSS that is concerned with the NHS). Now clearly this is just a joke . . . but there is no doubt that the bureaucracy does have close and important links with the concerned pressure groups and that some of these will have closer access and more apparent influence than others.

As I suggested in Chapter 1, there may also develop close links between the department and the Commons committee closely involved with overseeing it. In the same way, there may develop shared interests between departments and pressure groups. There are dangers associated with this, perhaps most notably the disparity of power and influence between the 'producers' and 'consumers' of medical care. If the doctors have developed a much closer link with their government department than other groups with an interest in health policy they will have a major input in determining perception of the parameters of the possible and the ideology of the department. It may be that the doctors' pressure group does not represent all the opinions and interests of the profession. It is a mistake to view medicine as a monolith. As well as differences of opinion, there are some major structural differences built in (between consultants and junior hospital doctors, for example) and there has also always been evident a culture of opposition to the dominant form of medicine and health planning from within medicine itself.

Steve Watkins (1987) offers an analysis of input of doctors to the policy-making process at the level of contact with the bureaucracy. The major institutions of the medical profession that operate at national level are the General Medical Council (GMC), the British Medical Association (BMA), the Royal Colleges and the protection societies (the Medical Defence Union, the Medical Protection Society and the Medical and Dental Defence Union of Scotland). In terms of their importance in this part of the policy-making process it is the Royal Colleges and the BMA that we need to be most concerned with. The Royal Colleges played an important role in the establishment of the NHS and the history of the tactics Bevan used to recruit their support for his proposed service provide a fascinating study of a pressure-group–politician interaction (Foot 1975). Then, as often thereafter, they seemed to see their interests as separate from those of the BMA. Bevan sought to make use of this important split which reflected a fundamental difference in priority between specialists employed in the hospital service and general practitioners whose voice was of particular importance in the BMA.

Today the Royal Colleges are responsible for the training of specialists, for setting specialist examinations and issuing certificates of accreditation which declare individuals suitable for consultant appointments. They are consulted by the government about professional matters and sit on joint committees with the BMA – the Joint Consultative Committee in the case of the hospital service; the more obviously named Community Medicine Consultative Committee; and the General Medical Services Committee/ Royal College of General Practice Joint Committee in the case of general practice.

The BMA's position *vis-à-vis* representation and negotiation is slightly complicated by the existence of 'craft committees' which are the bodies recognized as having the right to negotiate for doctors. These represent all doctors and not just members of the BMA, though they operate under the broad ambit of the BMA. About 70 per cent of doctors are members of the BMA, though the proportion was as low as 50 per cent in the mid-1970s. The craft committees include ones for general medical services; hospital junior staff; the Central Committee for Hospital Medical Services; the Central Committee for Community Medicine and Community Health; and the Medical Academic Staffs Committee.

Both the Royal Colleges and the BMA have, through their committee structure, very strong links with the DHSS. There may be times when the government would want to appeal over the heads of this structure on a specific issue but it seems to have great difficulty doing this. Specifically on the issue of private practice the Medical Practitioners Union advised the then Labour government in 1975 to offer a substantially increased differential to those consultants who worked full-time for the NHS and to offer that, if need be, over the heads of the profession's leaders. Both the advice on content and that on procedure were ignored. Instead the government decided to pursue the question of pay beds. The profession saw this as an attack on its economic interests and determined to fight it. The result was a settlement which Watkins (1987, p. 88) describes as 'botched . . . the anti-private practice cause was set back twenty years'. It is an episode worth looking at in some more detail because it did reveal the very particular lines consultation is forced along when the formal channels are used. It also addresses the more theoretical point of bureaucracies as inhibitors of radical change.

Private practice has always operated with twin motives on the part of the practitioners: one financial – it certainly can be a lucrative source of income outside, and in addition to, NHS salaries – and the other ideological. This ideology links a reluctance to give the state a monopoly on health care with a continuing, and allied, concern to preserve an area of professional independence. The opportunity for private practice varies according to the specialism and seniority of the doctor and to the part of the country in which he or she practices. Its popularity and the rationalisations doctors use to support it have also changed over time.

Consultants came into the NHS determined to preserve the tradition of private practice but until the mid-1970s seemed imperceptibly to shift towards a situation in which they obtained, and appeared happy to obtain, the majority of their work and income from the NHS. They were concerned with pay and conditions of service but the direction of their concern was to improve both within the framework of the NHS. The history of the NHS includes many road to Damascus conversions as an increasing number of parties incorporated support of the NHS into their *raison d'être*, decided that it was *their* NHS and discovered anyway that they were its true preservers/supporters (the Conservative Party, the Liberals and assorted medical pressure groups have made such claims). Watkins (1987, p. 88) suggests that among 'the [medical] profession's leadership the attachment to private practice was greater, since the leadership have a greater emotional attachment to the mythology of the profession and take longer to catch up with its changing moods'. This is an interesting comment both because it points to the 'mistakes' in government tactics which revitalized interest in private practice and because it illustrates some of the politics of bureaucracy, in this case the bureaucracy of the Royal Colleges and the BMA.

If the profession's leaders acted as the culture carriers the events of 1975 meant that both in their ideological commitment and, increasingly, in their practical activity private practice was pushed back to a position of importance. The settlement reached was that pay beds were to go, gradually, and in return the differential between consultants who worked entirely for the NHS and consultants who worked also in private practice was reduced from two-elevenths of salary to one-eleventh. Consultants could earn up to 10 per cent of their income from private practice without incurring a penalty. In effect, this was not just licensing a pay increase for some but making it much more likely that increasing numbers of consultants would become involved in private practice. That was 1975 – since then the whole area of private practice has been something that specific government policies have further supported and stimulated.

The links between the BMA and the DHSS do suggest the possibility of the development of 'clientism' (Richardson and Jordan 1979, p. 55), a situation where the relationship becomes so close that shared priorities develop between the inside and outside interests. The boundary between the group and the government becomes indistinct. This causes problems for anyone, or any group, wishing to contribute to the policy-making process but not enjoying this access.

There are very many other bodies with a concern in health and illness. Some represent consumers, or potential consumers, of services. Some are, at least in part, funded by the government. Groups like Age Concern and MIND have a broad range of interests and wish to have their opinion heard on many issues. Other groups have a more specific area of concern and may be in competition with others operating in the same area: for example, groups concerned with the law on abortion include the Society for the Protection of the Unborn Child, the Abortion Law Reform Association and LIFE. Although these groups can be important and influential, they are not as integrated into the bureaucracy as the groups representing doctors and so often pursue their attempts to influence policy via channels outside the DHSS. They may make considerable attempts at influencing public opinion, hence bringing pressure to bear via Parliament as well as offering the sort of expert advice that they hope will be found welcome by ministers and Civil Servants. Some have managed to gain posts within the legislature: for example, MIND's Secretary, Tony Smyth, acted as Secretary to the all-party parliamentary committee that oversees the mental health services.

These pressure groups act as a potential countervailing force to the doctor–DHSS axis. As such they draw our attention to issues that have been important in political science. Is the best description of the political power structure one of a power elite or is it better described using pluralist theory? Pluralist theory argues that power in Western industrial societies is widely distributed amongst different groups, sources of power are distributed non-cumulatively, as are money, information and expertise (Dahl 1961). A contrary theory has been built around an analysis of just how open to group influences the British system is. This analysis would have us believe that pluralism has given way to corporatism in which some groups are much stronger than others. In particular Cawson (1982) argues that 'the pressure group world is not fluid and competitive, but hierarchical, stratified and inegalitarian'. Organizations such as the BMA are well placed because of their 'strategic location in society'. Cawson argues that there is a coexistence of pluralism and corporatism. The doctors are snug in their corporate liaison with the government via the DHSS and other groups like Age Concern operate in a more casual and competitive environment.

This does indeed sound convincing and necessitates a reworking of pluralism. It is hard to see how you can have a little bit of pluralism. Pluralism in one area, with its varying alliances and fluctuating fortunes, is more likely. It is also a model that requires comparison of the public and private worlds of political negotiation. The doctors are likely to be involved in private negotiations within the machinery of the bureaucracy while the other pressure groups have to make their position known through public debate. The changing relationship of public and private discourses on health policy offers a useful way of assessing the fortunes of competing interests and of the permeability of the bureaucracy to private influence.

The reality of doctor power within the executive is a subject of particular relevance when seeking to evaluate the impact of managerialism, particularly following the Griffiths reforms (DHSS 1983a). There appears a determined effort to question some of the dominant planning assumptions in health and to rework the ideology of planning to centre on the more overt acceptance of the primacy of the economic. It may be that such a primacy has always existed, but it has not always been acknowledged. It will be a subject of analysis in what follows but here I will look briefly at the specific response of the medical profession to NHS cuts. One writer (Neale 1983) makes the connection nicely when he says that the increasing emphasis on managerialism in the NHS can be attributed to an attempt to reduce the influence of consultants so that cuts can be implemented. But it is a connection that needs to be researched, not just asserted. It must be located in the spectrum of change created because of conspiratorial machinations and change accruing, incrementally, from an already determined dynamic.

The arrival of managerialism as a potential counter-ideology, struggling for dominance with an established one, is perhaps the crucial contemporary issue to explore. It addresses all the questions of bureaucratic and professional power we have been looking at but also encourages us to reflect on the nature of history and change in the NHS and in public policy in general.

It may be that the nature of discourse in society is shifting away from the rationalist positivism epitomized by a social construction of medicine, although not evident when its detailed practice is examined (the element of the mystical, of faith, is still so central to the therapeutic encounter). This shift is towards a managerialism that has to be considered using different explanatory constructs. It may also lay claim to rationality and good sense but it likewise has an underlife, antecedents and impacts that require other forms of understanding.

If such a change is occurring then it might also relate to shifts in the broad historical paradigm either into a different – some say late, some last (depending on their optimism) – stage of capitalism. Others talk in terms of a shift from modernism to post-modernism and still others talk of yet another shift in the dominant form of discourse, neither better nor worse, neither higher nor lower, but typical of discontinuity, break and rupture. Conversely, perhaps nothing much has changed beyond a shift in the language of presentation. Managerialism may always have been evident. It may have been called something else but have manifested the same principles. Or it may now be just a spectre, nothing of substance, and the dominant ideology of health and of the NHS may be carrying on regardless.

In the official history of the BMA some of the changes and divisions in medicine are made clear when the authors say that

the NHS is popular with the public but not with the doctors.

Medicine and politics do not mix well. In the first half of its existence it was the general practitioners who found the most difficulty in living with socialised medicine, and in the second half, the chief problems and discontents have arisen in the hospital service and amongst hospital doctors (Grey-Turner and Sutherland 1982, p. 164).

But those discontents have not been such as to mobilize either the hospital doctors or the BMA against the NHS as such. Indeed, in its public pronouncements the BMA has taken a more active role of speaking in defence of the NHS. For example, in 1981 the Chairman of the annual representatives' meeting of the BMA made a speech at its conference defending the NHS and calling for more resources, and in 1984 a different chair referred specifically to 'problems with the Conservative government' (quoted in Watkins 1987, pp. 97–8). It is now not unusual for government statements on public expenditure to receive critical responses from the BMA, or for the BMA to conduct surveys about the effect of cuts on patient care. Further, and most notably in its work on the medical effects of nuclear war, the BMA (or at least sub-committees of it) defines its area of competence more broadly than the narrowly medical.

But all this opens is a space, a window of opportunity, for more radical practice. It is not the whole picture or even the dominant dynamic in a profession that, if it feels itself beleaguered, retreats to a narrow defence of individual financial gain, through private practice, and to a narrow specialism in emphasizing super-technologism – the gains that can be made by high-technology modern medicine. Doctors, as a profession, are increasingly (and increasingly because of the more stark choices that are now faced in Thatcherite Britain) in the position of having to choose between their professional interest and their class interest. Because the economic conditions of their labour are not uniform some will be able to identify their interests in oppositional terms and, because choice to act is not rigidly predetermined, some will choose to step outside the dominant definition of class interest. But most will not.

We should be wary of presenting too narrow a concentration on one part of the apparatus of the state. It would be a mistake to develop an atomized analysis. To obtain an accurate picture it is necessary to see the parts in their relationship and interaction, to see them dialectically. This is true in looking at the bureaucracy and pressure groups and helps to see the more than institutional ties that bind the doctors and the DHSS senior bureaucrats.

At the same time it is not legitimate to investigate these ties using only the methods of positivism and empiricism. Weber may have presented bureaucracy as the inevitable product of a social dynamic located in reason. But the use of reason both to determine the functioning and social role of the bureaucracy and to evaluate its effectiveness is akin to using a part of the debatable problematic to evaluate the very thing it emanates from. One must look outside the narrow confines of positivism and evaluate it critically and in action.

Bennis (1966), in presenting the complexities of bureaucracy, tells us that it 'is much easier to deplore than to describe'. The problem with much description is that it reads like the story of four men in a small room having to describe an elephant – one could only see its legs and described it as like a tree, one could only see its ears and thought it more like a sail, and so on. It is necessary to get some distance from it so that the whole can be seen all at once to realize what it is! I have been trying to get that distance but will conclude this brief examination of the NHS bureaucracy with a short description of the actual structure as it was evident within the DHSS.

The DHSS was a department of state that had been in existence since 1968, having emerged from that year of bureaucratic mergers out of a coming together of the ministries of Health and of Social Security. The Secretary of State was the political head, assisted by a Minister of Health responsible for that part of the department associated with the NHS. Although one department, there are separate administrative structures for health and personal social services and for social security. Indeed, in 1987 and 1988 the possibility of breaking up the DHSS and creating completely separate administrations was under discussion. This break-up finally happened in 1988 and will be discussed in Chapter 10.

In the early years of the NHS housing was within the remit of the Ministry and then was taken away. Then it was argued that health and housing were discrete areas requiring separate administrations. There were advantages and disadvantages to this. Joint planning was made much more difficult. For example, the integration of community health services with new housing developments did not take place. But having a less complex ministry did allow the political head to exercise more direction and control. Similar arguments are relevant to the DHSS. Beveridge was no doubt right that income maintenance was essential to a health service – and vice versa – but there had not been an emphasis on joint planning and the DHSS remained a huge and cumbersome department.

Between 1972 and the implementation of the Griffiths reforms the health side of the DHSS was split into four organizational divisions: one was concerned with personnel matters; one with finance, including negotiations with the Treasury; one with maintaining links with the health authorities; and the fourth with service development. The Griffiths Report (DHSS 1983a), in commenting on this structure, identified fragmentation at the centre and an absence of a sharp management focus. Many health administrators would have agreed with this, particularly in the division between maintaining links with the authorities and with service development – they might have identified it as a split between line management and planning. Further, the DHSS was not overseeing the operation of the service in the regions as effectively as Griffiths thought necessary. To overcome this weakness the Report recommended the establishment of a Health Services Supervisory Board and an NHS Management Board within the DHSS. The proposal was accepted by the Secretary of State and the Supervisory Board was set up in 1983 under his chairmanship.

The functions identified for this board were the determination of the purpose, objectives and direction of the NHS; appraisal of the overall budget and resource allocation; strategic decisions; and receiving reports on performance and other evaluations from within the NHS. The Management Board was to be responsible for planning and implementing policies approved by the Supervisory Board, giving leadership in the management of the NHS, controlling performance and achieving consistency and drive over the long term. The two boards would overlap in personnel only in so far as the chairman of the Management Board would also sit on the Supervisory Board, although it was expected that the Management Board would work 'under the direction of the Minister'. The Supervisory Board set up in 1983 had as members, in addition to the Secretary of State, other health ministers in the DHSS; the Permanent Secretary; the Chief Medical Officer; the Chief Nursing Officer and Roy Griffiths (Chairman of the Committee this new structure emanated from). The Management Board, chaired by an 'outside appointment', would include individuals with responsibility for personnel; finance; procurement; property; scientific and high-technology management; and service planning. The changes were designed to contribute to the identified aim in the Griffiths Report of establishing at the centre a coherent management process that would allow the setting of broad strategic objectives for the NHS and ensure that through appropriate planning and monitoring mechanisms these objectives were achieved. If there was a coherent management process then the Department could 'prune many of its existing activities' (DHSS 1983, p. 15).

From the outset it was clear that there was a need to examine what was meant by, and understood about, the relationship between planning and management. Another potential area for confusion was that between the development of a more interventionist centre and a wish to shift responsibilities onto the regions and districts. It was likely also that changes in management and planning would affect accountability and hence call into question some of the established relationships both with Parliament and regional and district health authority members.

The first chairman of the NHS Management Board was Victor Paige, who had previously worked in industry, at the National Freight Corporation and the Port of London. His three-year appointment was initially greeted with some criticism because of his lack of experience in health, although a reading of the Griffiths Report would have stopped anyone assuming that was necessary for a chairman. The *Health and Social Service Journal* (*HSSJ*, 10 January 1985, p. 36) somewhat coyly reported that there was some suspicion that he was not heavyweight enough (it is uncertain what list of heavyweights they had in mind) and that his appointment might be indicative of the DHSS's attempting to reduce the importance of the Management Board and its chairman from the central role envisaged in the Griffiths Report (see DHSS 1983a, para 4, p. 4). They were posing as a new problematic a potential area of dispute between the Board and the established departmental culture. The first things Victor Paige said to the press did sound consistent with a culture of 'new realism'. He spoke of the primacy of the patient, of participative management and of the need to learn from business that sometimes decisions have to be made based on incomplete evidence (*HSSJ*, 24 January 1985, p. 94).

The response of the DHSS to the introduction of general management has officially been that it is a process that has gone relatively smoothly. But from the outset there was speculation that senior officials in the DHSS were conspiring to protect their own position and effectively nullifying the proper installation of the general management function, at least at the top level (Halpern 1985, p. 248). In fact the changes that a proper implementation of the Griffiths reforms would necessitate appear fundamental. The previous management structure, incidentally the result of a package designed in the early 1970s by management consultants McKinsey and Co., appeared strongly biased towards various client groups, the opposite of the Griffiths prescription. But critics of the introduction of an apparently more straightforward system might point to the reality of complexity in the service. Perhaps a simplified organization and management structure might lose some of the possibilities for identifying the interconnections between different parts of the NHS's activities and also the relationship between political and administrative needs. This criticism sees the Griffiths changes as imposing an inappropriate mechanistic model on an organic organizational structure. It did not take long after the introduction of the Griffiths reforms for NHS administrators to begin to talk wistfully about consensus management as 'not that bad' and 'a system that just wasn't given enough time to work properly'.

I will, at this point, use three examples to illustrate some of the areas of concern following the acceptance of the Griffiths recommendations. First, in the policy area of community care we can see how the Griffiths changes would affect very many parts of the NHS. All these separate interests and perspectives could be represented at some point in the old structure. One can envisage very many of the different interest groupings having at least some point of access to the debate about community care. Within such an organizational structure two possibilities exist. One is that this multiplicity of interest would mean no clear picture and that no effective operational policy would emerge. The other is that a simplified management structure would mean no clear picture and that no effective operational policy would emerge! The same result for different reasons, one because of too much complexity the other because of too much simplicity.

Second, there may be a problem in reconciling the two functions of the DHSS Civil Servants in serving the Secretary of State politically and in administering the services of the DHSS. For example, the issue of accountability may give rise to areas of potential conflict. Before Griffiths, in 1982, a system of accountability reviews was set up. Regions became managerially accountable to the Secretary of State. Each region would agree to certain objectives and the extent to which these were achieved was the subject of review. A similar process was introduced by regions for districts and, following Griffiths, a similar process will be extended to units. Review offers the possibility to assess both objectives and achievement. It may be that a region, district or unit is not meeting its targets and that this is indicative of management shortcomings. But it can also indicate inappropriately set and inadequately resourced targets. Traditionally the politician has identified targets as vaguely as possible – 'we will improve community care', for example. This means that with the use of some selective examples and an 'economical way with the truth' Civil Servants and ministers have been able to minimize political damage from bad performance in their areas of responsibility. If the Griffiths review system is to work there will need to be much more specific targets, with a corresponding increase in political risk.

The third area of difficulty lies in clarifying the relationship between the Secretary of State (or Minister), the DHSS, and the regions and districts. We are presented with a confusing picture in which it seems there is no line-management responsibility between the management boards and the NHS in the regions and districts. The Management Board, if it was to do what Griffiths had wanted, would need to have access to the constituent parts of the NHS in such a way as to permit long-term direction, give leadership and so achieve consistency. The first and third of these considerations would not necessarily be in harmony with the political interests of the secretary of state or minister – in the long term, after all, a person is out of office! This sets up the possibility of the Management Board seeking to act in ways that would set it in opposition to the minister. This is in addition to the continuing potential for opposition with the previously established DHSS structure.

Perhaps the biggest danger to the success of the Griffiths changes within the DHSS is that the Management Board becomes just another part of the Department. Halpern (1985, p. 249) describes 'Mr. Paige in the next office along from his fellow second permanent secretary, the chief medical officer, surrounded by the same pot plants and the same civil servants'. It is this possibility of incorporation that must be a major feature of any review of the work of the Board. Paige's appointment on a short fixed-term contract might have been considered as a way of insuring against this but it has to be asked whom the chairman must please to gain reappointment.

The dilemma might be more specifically identified if we look at the difference between what is considered as necessary for good management and what some senior Civil Servants have described as the essence of their job. Central to the senior Civil Servant's function is offering protection to the minister. It does appear that Civil Servants who spend time with ministers and do this part of the job well are destined for even higher office (or perhaps it is that those destined for high office are first placed in close proximity to ministers for a time). Such officers are also good at protecting themselves and keeping well out of the spotlight. But there are occasional lapses. Dr William Plowden, now Director of the Royal Institute of Public Administration but a former Civil Servant, said in a recent speech that most officials see themselves as the confidential advisers of ministers rather than the managers of activities; they look up, not down. Jobs which involve the management of activities command very low prestige, even though they may involve control over very large resources. Further, to become more effective Civil Servants risk having to pay the price of becoming personally and publicly more accountable for their own decisions (Halpern 1985, p. 250).

I will return to the broader issues but cannot let this observation pass without linking it with Niskanen's model. It presents an analysis of motivation and activity which undermines the budget-maximization approach for bureaucratic development. It is an argument that links well with Weber's model, as adapted to recognize the limitations on initiative and hence the essential conservatism of such a regime.

Halpern presents two more illustrative examples, one in the area of costs and cuts and the other concerning the gap between planning and management. He cites a memorandum to the Treasury from the DHSS which pointed to the increased cost of new forms of treatment being about 0.5 per cent of current annual spending. At the same time the practice of discharging people earlier from hospital would save about 0.5 per cent a year. So the one could offset the other. (This was in a memorandum to the Treasury, after all, and must have been reassuring to them – they had already included a figure for new technologies in a calculation of annual cost increases.) This sort of neat rationalism reads like a commodification in which ends appear overwhelmed by a consideration of means and all gets subsumed under a neat accountancy.

Secondly, we must understand planning and the implementation of policy as integrated activities, for example in an area like community care. But every government has supported this policy since the early 1970s and very few old psychiatric hospitals have been closed. Those people who have been discharged have been sent, often, to inadequate alternatives. Now it may be that the policy was only sophistry, that there was never any real intention. It may be that it is a policy that was intended but never understood in its implications and so the gap between decision and action was never bridged. It may be that it was a policy more important as a manifestation of a power struggle within the interest groups constellation that contributes to policy-making in health. Or it may have epitomized an attempt to reconstruct the dominant ideology. If it is the last of these then, indeed, it should be understood as a rhetorical struggle – a problem in discourse and not to do with its apparent subject. Or if such a policy was really intended it may be that the abilities of the DHSS and of Civil Servants as managers were not adequate to put it into effect. Or it may have been all of these, but it certainly illustrates a massive gap between planning and implementation.

The Griffiths proposals do appear to attempt to address some of these issues, albeit still within the narrow confines of a conventional definition of health and ill-health. But to succeed will require a place where the political demands that are made on the NHS are converted into workable management objectives. That place could be the Management Board. But such changes do not seem easy, in the short term at least. By 1987 there was still much discussion on the need to resolve the differences and conflicts involved in the relationship between managers, the government and Civil Servants. The Health Minister, Tony Newton, identified the major objective of the NHS Management Board as converting the government's aspirations into management reality. But if they do this they risk a temptation to collude with the pretence of delivering the undeliverable, or of being unduly preoccupied with reacting to short-term political crisis.

Newton was saying that NHS management cannot be divorced from politics (*HSSJ*, 12 March 1987). But this was not the only unresolved issue: there was still a problem in separating administration and management. This was evident in the identified problem of DHSS officials telephoning NHS managers when they were anxious about a particular decision or problem they perceived that manager as having. In such situations Civil Servants act in the tried and tested way of wishing to protect their political masters from embarrassment. But this does interfere with managers' sense of independence of movement.

A pattern of communication outside the formally acknowledged has been evident throughout the Thatcher government. It makes it important in an analysis of planning and policy-making to look at the 'private' discourse, that occurring within the formal structure, and the 'public', that conveyed from one part of the structure to another via an external agency – usually the media. Early in Thatcher's first term as Prime Minister, for example, Webb and Wistow (1982, p. 32) identified a process of 'government by ministerial speech'. This was most evident in the area of personal social services but also touched health policy. Commenting on 1979–80, they suggest that this practice might have been a reflection of 'a temporary policy and administrative vacuum which existed until the department developed programmes and instruments more consistent with its minister's philosophy of governance'. But an alternative explanation might point to the contradictions evident within the policy itself which may explain why different messages were transmitted in different media. The Secretary of State, Patrick Jenkin, was speaking about a policy based on disengagement: 'It is the government's firm policy that detailed planning and management of resources are best left to those on the spot who know local needs and priorities' (DHSS Press Notice 80/201, 5 August 1980). But at the same time there was an evident increase in attention to the detail of policy in government speeches. It was not just this difference between the words used in internal communication from the DHSS to the authorities and the public practice of interventionism. In its legislative and administrative programme there were also examples of the government taking more control. The centre was being enhanced and this was being achieved particularly by eroding the sphere of local government activity and autonomy. An early example was the tighter controls on local government spending introduced in the Local Government Finance (No 2) Bill which appeared to sit oddly alongside the declared intention of increased local autonomy. There are many more examples but in health the most interesting is the argument that the Griffiths reforms are, in practice, producing a considerably more centralized service despite the rhetoric of devolving responsibility.

An interesting development arising out of shifts to a policy orientated towards community care for the mentally ill and the mentally handicapped is that there is evident an increasing amount of co-operation between health districts and local authorities. This co-operation is facilitated, in the main, by a use of health authority funds and appears to be one of the few areas in which an expansion of local government activity is apparent in a political climate where its services and its record are usually under considerable critical pressure. It is no wonder that the local authorities, in the main, welcome these approaches from the NHS.

A further example of the extent of central involvement in local health district activity lies in the work of the Inter Regional Secretariat. This is a body made up of 28 NHS chairmen and managers and has been called, among other things, 'the NHS's most powerful quango' and the Secretary of State's 'secret society'. Its role is to facilitate communication between ministers and the Management Board, on the one hand, and the NHS, on the other. It developed out of a wish to involve regional officers more closely with the DHSS. The aim, ostensibly, was to effect a reduction in the volume of communication so that appropriate attention could be paid to the most essential items. But in practice it appeared to provide a conduit for the transmission of information from the centre and, as such, to increase the power of regions over districts and, in turn, of the centre over the regions. It facilitates communication rather than advises on procedure and it is a predominantly one-way communication. The Secretariat briefs regional chairmen on all current issues and separately briefs regional general managers. It seeks to 'form a consensus view' from the regions to be taken to the Management Board and the ministers. Critics of the Secretariat say that in ironing out 'lumps and bumps' it is protecting the Board and the Minister from the diversity of views and problems in the regions (Allenway 1987, p. 762). As such it is creating a false consensus and structuring debate in such a way as to aid the centralizing tendencies present in post-Griffiths practice. The Secretariat's budget is not made known and its deliberations are considered confidential.

The Secretariat exists independently of the National Association of Health Authorities (NAHA), a body the Secretary of the Inter Regional Secretariat, David Blyth, calls a 'trade association'. The NAHA expresses NHS views to ministers and Civil Servants, investigates specific issues and problems and maintains links with the Press and Parliament. It has a staff of nine and, in 1984, a budget of £150,000 (Ham 1985, p. 108). Barbara Castle had attended the first annual conference of the NAHA and there had encouraged the NAHA to become a 'pressure group for the NHS' (Castle 1980, p. 459). But if it is a pressure group it is operating in an environment where it has to compete alongside the Secretariat. In contrast to Barbara Castle's pressure group, Norman Fowler described regional chairmen acting as a 'health cabinet' (House of Commons Social Services Committee 1984, p. 165) and there certainly is a lot of difference between the impact of a pressure group and of a cabinet!

It is interesting to speculate about the understanding of 'consensus' as it is used to describe the operation of the Secretariat. Consensus can be something reached after a long period of mutual exchange and compromise or it can be something that is agreed to because no other course appears viable. It can be created or imposed. Perhaps Norman Fowler's experience of the Cabinet is more consistent with the latter than the former model, that is, the Cabinet is somewhere where you are told what you will do and you agree. Not only do you agree but you discover that you always agreed anyway.

Griffiths reforms will also have an impact on the access of pressure groups to the decision-making process. If such an impact can be measured in the degree of dislike expressed by doctors then it would seem to be creating a definite change. At the BMA Annual Conference in 1987 the doctors seemed unanimous in their dislike of the new management. The consultants' leader, Paddy Ross, spoke of 'insensitive and incompetent management' and warned that services to patients would improve only in those units where managers work with consultants and not against them.

The spirit of this comment reverses the expectation of Griffiths which was that consultants should work with managers. The leader of the junior hospital doctors, Peter Hawker, talked of the 'clump of hobnail boots of managers in the corridors of power' and of 'blitzkriegs against junior staff'. The Conference passed resolutions opposing the principle of doctors being made accountable to non-medical managers and emphasizing that doctors are professionally accountable to the General Medical Council and only managerially accountable, if so contracted, for specific managerial jobs ('Doctors Despair of Management' *HSSJ*, 9 July 1987).

3   The Legislature

The theoretical position of the minister responsible to the legislature and the legislature voting funds to the NHS puts Parliament at the heart of policy-making in health. But in reality executive government and executive power mean that scrutiny and representation are perhaps the two most important features of Parliament's role. The first is most effectively located in the committee structure. The second is most important in adding to the NHS an air of legitimacy rather than in fundamentally shaping it. But as the symbolic achievement of the NHS, its contribution to a dominant ideology, is of central importance and at times more important than what it actually does, this legitimating function is worthy of study.

In a valuable study of Parliament and health policy between 1970 and 1975 Ingle and Tether (1981, p. 1) make the following observation about representation and legitimation,

> The process of representation has to do basically with the transcription of the recommendations of experts into the kinds of symbols which the informed but non-expert layman will understand and will be able to pass judgement on. This passing of judgement is referred to in constitutional language as legitimising.

If this is so then the clarity and honesty with which the recommendations are presented, debated and communicated is crucial. It is also important to identify whether individual members' differences of opinion as to the role of parliamentarians are of importance or whether the key issue is the overall stance of the institution.

When looking at the contribution of individual parliamentarians there are two features to identify. The first is the position of the MP *vis-à-vis* the dominant power structure. The second is the perception the MP has of his or her own role. Some MPs will have individual assumptive worlds that conform closely with the dominant belief system, while those of others will diverge significantly from it (Young 1977, p. 3). Each has to decide what part of these assumptive worlds should take precedence on any individual issue. This presents some of the same issues as those identified in the examination of the roles of the Secretary of State earlier. An MP will have conflicting personal agendas that usually centre on reconciling the demands of representing a constituency and therefore being subject to re-election, being a member of a party and subject to its favour in individual advancement, and having an individual philosophy that may at times not sit easily with the first two considerations.

Some issues will bring these considerations into acute conflict. For example, an MP may be in favour of cuts in public expenditure but wish to support the retention of a hospital threatened with closure in his or her constituency. Or again, party and pressure group interests may clash when an MP is also a doctor and proposed changes in practice are seen as infringing on the clinical independence of doctors. Or there may be a conflict when a moral belief and a party policy are at odds, as they might be in changes in abortion law, for example. Individual MPs are also in different positions in terms of closeness to the executive. The tactics of an MP who is also a minister and that of an Opposition back-bencher will clearly be different and the use they make of the platform of the House of Commons will reflect this.

A.H. Birch (1964) identified four different views on representation held by MPs. The first he termed 'deputational'; this is where an MP sees his or her function as to further the general good of all constituents. The second he termed 'ideological', here the MP sees himself or herself as mandated to implement policies on which he or she fought for election. The third, 'advocative', is the stance of the MP who sees his or her primary function as being to support particular interests. The fourth, 'custodial', describes the MP who sees him- or herself as a watchdog and as such essentially non-partisan. These stances may change from time to time and from issue to issue but the four of them together provide a framework for the analysis of the role of MPs in making and overseeing health policy.

Ingle and Tether (1981, p. 153) identify each of these types of stance taken by MPs but locate them in an overall analysis that concludes that, 'as far as health in the period 1970–5 was concerned, Parliament's ability to influence the policies of the government was minimal'. Further, its capacity to scrutinize policy and its application and to modify it where necessary was largely absent. It was lost in both the party system and in a system dominated by the executive. Even the opportunity the existence of Parliament affords to MPs to take advantage of informal contact with ministers and so influence policy is 'in no way comparable to the influence exerted by interest groups and civil servants in the pre-legislative process' (Ingle and Tether 1981, p. 155).

Before moving on to consider the importance of these findings for the role of Parliament as legitimator, I will look in a little more detail at the kinds of area and decision on which Ingle and Tether based their conclusions. Looking at the number of column inches devoted to the second reading debate on the Bill which later became the National Health Reorganization Act 1973, they found that 36 per cent of the time spent was taken up with partisan or ideological input, custodial input accounted for 21 per cent, deputational for 23 per cent, and advocative for 20 per cent. They could find nothing to convince them that any sort of intervention was useful, or that one sort was more effective than another.

There is a Fabian argument that democracy is best judged by its actions and its capacity to maximize welfare. If the government of the day acts efficiently to make welfare generally available, then it is acting democratically because it is reflecting some sort of general will. It may be then that the government was not listening to the sectional interests of MPs because it represented a broader consensus and because it had got its legislation right. But the truth was the reorganization of 1974 was welcomed by almost nobody when it was seen in operation. Indeed, a Royal Commission was soon established with very wide frames of reference to review, among other things, structure. This was legislation in need of considerable scrutiny and modification. It did not get it. Either the scrutiny was not evident or it was not effective in creating modifications.

It was possible to see MPs following up constituents' complaints and pursuing items of local interest, even if this meant criticizing the government. There was the possibility of scrutinizing Civil Servants using the Parliamentary question and seeking an adjournment debate. These things were done but their effect, as analysed by Ingle and Tether, was not as effective in achieving any sort of redress as the more straightforward move of contacting the Press! Adjournment debates were ranked high by MPs in terms of their efficacy in getting issues raised and alerting the government to things going wrong. While it is hard to identify specific cases of redress obtained, it may be that raising such issues does help ensure that the same kinds of problem do not arise again. The Aztecs used to sacrifice to the sun every night, believing that if they did not then the sun would not return next day. The stakes were too high to experiment by one day not doing it to see if the feared result would, in fact, occur. Parliament is a bit like that. MPs go on asking questions, talking in debates, canvassing support and contacting ministers, often with no apparent result. But they fear that if they stopped then things would get worse. Maybe a better analogy is that of the boy with his finger in the dyke! Jeremy Seabrook argues that traditionally parliamentarians have displayed 'histrionic skills' deployed in the interests of concealment and deception. He warns that they cannot safeguard freedoms but do their best to 'conjure such threats out of sight' (Guardian, 9 September 1987).

Various committees of the House have a relevance in regard to health policy. The style of select committees, as opposed to standing committees, is the first point to make. The former operate with more deliberative process and employ inquisitorial techniques. It is an approach that was recognized by a 1978 committee on procedure in the Commons as being more effective. This would certainly appear to be an accurate assessment when it is contrasted with descriptions of what goes on in standing committees. In the 1960s Richard Crossman described the whole Standing Committee system as 'insane'. He asked: 'What is the sense of working line by line through each clause when in many cases there is no one there who understands what they mean . . . there is no committee work, just formal speech making' (Crossman 1977). The same committee structure was subject, in 1987, to criticism by Lord Whitelaw, Conservative leader in the House of Lords. He dismissed the standing committees as no more than rubber stamps because each had a built-in government majority. The party representation on these committees replicated the Conservatives' overall parliamentary majority (at that time 101 MPs), so that each committee had a built-in government majority of between six and eight. The committees had little expectation of changing the substance of a Bill. It was rare for either a minister's recommendations to be overruled or for an Opposition amendment to be accepted.

> The Minister, whose detailed understanding of the issues in a Bill is often less than complete, has to rely on his civil servants. He relies more on his officials than on his backbenchers who, if not overtly troublesome, are rarely more than lobby fodder and use most of their time to catch up on correspondence (*Guardian*, 9 February 1988).

Opposition MPs rely on outside bodies, including pressure groups, to mirror the specialist service the minister gets from Civil Servants. Members of the Opposition do not often act in concert to make a determined attack on a Bill but rather seek to embarrass the government, highlight the 'real intention' in the Bill, clarify an issue or placate an outside interest or party supporter. In contrast, the government's intention seems to be to get the Bill through the committee as intact and as quickly as possible.

The House of Commons Committee of Public Accounts has often intervened in the area of NHS finance. Many of its comments have appeared both valuable and influential, for example its findings on financial controls of hospitals and on the hospital building programme (House of Commons Committee of Public Accounts 1988a). But this Committee does not appear to have an impact on the central issues within its apparent sphere of competence, for example in a scrutiny of the cost effectiveness of overall health programmes (House of Commons

Committee of Public Accounts 1988b). Like all committees, it becomes axiomatic that they are effective when what they suggest is accepted by the government. But a high level of acceptance can be achieved if they aim only to change the detail, or if they make recommendations consistent with the spirit and intention of the original Bill. Government policy and public expenditure are subject to scrutiny but the adjustments achieved are minor and not at all sufficient to meet some aspiration of parliamentary control over policy or expenditure. They are not enough to meet the claims, or aspirations, of some of those who present this Committee as more powerful than it is. But what is important to appreciate is that, given the immensity of the whole governmental undertaking, small changes in the overall scheme of things can profoundly improve an individual's experience of the impact of legislation and spending. Perhaps it is the claims and not the achievement of this Committee that are at fault.

The Social Services Committee is that body in the House which formally corresponds in its brief with the work carried out under the aegis of the DHSS. It carries out a number of inquiries into, and reviews of, the work of the NHS. Some of these are very specific and are usually in response to a change in government policy in a related area, for example the effect of cuts in university spending on medical services. But the Committee can also look at areas of general concern, such as the incidence of perinatal and neo-natal mortality. Further, it can consider more far-reaching issues, for example the organization and practice of health care. It might look at the Griffiths changes or at an area like community care (Ham 1985, p. 86).

The findings of the Committee and its recommendations do not have to be accepted by the government. Indeed, the call for more resources to be spent on child health and maternity services, which followed the Committee's research into perinatal and neo-natal mortality, was rejected by the government. Nevertheless Ham (1985, p. 87) concludes that the

committees create a more informed House of Commons, force departments to account for their actions, submit ministers to a level of questioning not possible on the floor of the House, and help to put items on the agenda for discussion. Furthermore, at a time when the role and influence of individual MPs have come into question, the committees have given MPs useful and often satisfying work to do.

When one puts this analysis alongside the more sceptical one of Ingle and Tether, one might want to identify the role of MPs as being the power to stop things the executive might have considered doing if the legislature were not there in the first place, but not to intervene once the executive has decided upon something. Such an argument is reminiscent of Steven Lukes's (1974) views on the nature of power. He argues that studies have been too preoccupied with the more visible dimensions of power relations, for example the individual's behaviour in decision-making on issues where there is an observable conflict of preferences. He wishes to present another, less visible, dimension of power operating through collective forces and social arrangements to suppress potential issues and avert conflict. Power is related to both the capacity to do something and the capacity to stop something being done. In the parliamentary context, it may be that committees and general debate in the House have little impact *vis-à-vis* visible dimensions of power but may be important both in the less visible and in the generation of a sense of legitimacy.

Many MPs grow very disillusioned with the role they have to adopt. Paul Rose, an MP in the 1974–9 Parliament who decided not to stand for re-election, pointed to the 'licensed jester [being] permitted but the men with ideas and integrity . . . [being] either smothered in a messy system of group responsibility or blotted out' (Ingle and Tether 1981, p. 156). There are activities in every profession which its practitioners carry out knowing that they are at odds with the aims of the profession. I am a lecturer and am familiar with an impressive body of educational research which informs me that lectures are a very bad way of communicating information. Yet I continue to lecture. Perhaps the research does not apply to me, I think, because of my abilities or the idiosyncrasies of my style. Or I tell myself that other teaching methods also have their problems. But I know that I lecture for reasons other than pedagogic ones, reasons that are more to do with my status and with a particular construction of proper behaviour. The MP, I believe, is in an analogous position.

PART II

The Public Presentation of Health Policy

4   The Changing Structure of Health Care

From looking at the formal structure of policy-making in the executive and legislature I will now move on to a consideration of the communication of ideas and information around health policy. I intend to look at some of the actual issues that have been most evident in the period from 1984 until September 1987. The Griffiths Report (DHSS 1983a) came out in October 1983, so that by the start of 1984 its implications were being considered. September 1987 saw a major policy speech, from a new Secretary of State, John Moore, which provided little new but did reiterate some important key points in developing Conservative policy.

News reported in these years was voluminous. Each day the Press carried issues that related to the NHS either directly or tangentially. But the dominant issues have remained consistent. I will categorize them under four main headings: items concerned with the changing structure of health services; items relating to public expenditure and cuts in services (these either concentrate on general issues of finance or on specific instances where a hospital or service is believed to be under threat); privatization; and general policy on health related neither directly to structure nor to cuts, though often linked with one or both of these. Such issues link with broad political concerns and I will complete this section by looking at the 1987 general election to illustrate this. My survey of news stories is not comprehensive, though it does cover the main issues as identified in the press. My stance reflects a belief that in these troubled *Times* the *Guardian* became the paper of record for health and social services. In presenting them I am not suggesting these were the issues of either most immediate importance or of lasting concern.

I will offer a commentary that contrasts what is presented with the important issues as I, and other non-journalist commentators, have assessed them during this period. I am seeking to compare the public debate on health with that process of policy-making that occurs in the more private interchange within the structure of government. In doing this it becomes possible to make a more accurate assessment of the real distribution of power and the real nature of change within the system. Are MPs really part of the public debate or do they have some sort of access to the private? Do changes in governmental ideology and the introduction of new management ideas mean that pressure groups find the usual private channels closed and have to enter the more fluid public realm? Further, a concern of this work is to identify the nature of communication and its distortions. To pursue these agendas, despite its drawbacks, the following impressionistic review is useful.

In 1984 the British Medical Association (BMA), which has fought consistently against 'outside' interference, made it clear to all concerned, and particularly to Secretary of State Norman Fowler, that it would neither accept nor co-operate with plans to appoint 'super-executives' to run health authorities. In a letter sent by Mr Anthony Grabham, chairman of the BMA Council, to the Secretary of State and released to the Press on 11 January 1984 they argued that their reading of the Griffiths Report's (DHSS 1983a) proposals was that 'a somewhat autocratic executive manager' would take over. While this might be necessary and desirable in trade and commerce, it argued, it has no place in a health service which depends upon a number of caring professions working together.

This BMA statement was issued at the end of the time period set aside for consultation on the Griffiths proposals. It coincided with opposition that was also being expressed by some health authorities. One suggestion, made by district medical officers, was that the appointment of executives ought to be optional and that, where management was working well, authorities ought to be left alone to make their own arrangements. The West Midlands Regional Health Authority warned that imposing these changes on health authorities would do more harm than good and the Association of Nurse Administrators believed that the 'imposition of an industrial model of accountability on a service concerned with patient/client care is a cause for deep concern'. Michael Meacher, for the Labour Party, saw the proposed new management structure as being something the government was going to impose because it would facilitate the implementation of its 'destructive policies' with least resistance (*Guardian*, 11 January 1984).

Such reactions exhibit a range of justifiable concerns and professional misgivings. Some seemed closely related to the specific suggestions of Griffiths, while others stemmed from a generalized concern that another major reorganization of health services was the least desirable policy. Some objections to Griffiths were marked by a concern that the reforms would work and some that they would not!

It did appear that Griffiths was offering more than just a route to making savings, although, in itself, that had proved difficult enough. In 1982 a series of Rayner scrutinies was commissioned. These were to be 'ninety day business inspired exercises in the art of cutting red tape to produce near enough instant reports on how costs could be cut, bureaucracy disposed of, and money saved' (*The Times*, 20 February 1984). By the time the Griffiths report was being discussed ten Rayner scrutinies had been started, but none had reported. This completion rate was an example of business-type efficiency that brought some pleasure to NHS administrators. One of the problems with the Rayner scrutinies was that although they did offer specific suggestions, these, if acted upon, would have repercussions in areas that would not have been considered. They might be unwelcome to some specific interests or they might precipitate changes considered politically damaging. For example, a scrutiny of the provision of nurses' and doctors' homes suggested selling off much of the property and so releasing, for other NHS use, much needed capital. Money raised from these sales could be used to provide assisted mortgages and possibly subsidized rents, which the scrutiny suggested would be in the interests of staff. The general quality of much of the housing to be disposed of was very poor, though its city-centre location would make it desirable in the property market. But the scrutiny's recommendations, if implemented, would have added to an array of charges then current of asset-stripping in the NHS. Financial logic was superseded by political judgement and the recommendations were put to one side.

It has been a feature of recent policy that such suggestions reappear when they are not considered so politically sensitive or when the government does not feel so vulnerable. In this case we will see them reappear in a way that clearly remains asset-stripping. The rhetoric may be of efficiency and business sense but it is difficult to argue for anything other than the primacy of the political in short-term tactical decision-making.

Another Rayner scrutiny looked at staff advertising. It suggested cost-cutting by direct advertising rather than placing advertisements in commercial journals. It was a suggestion on which the journals, who draw heavily on job advertisement income, were not keen. Here the government would have been seen as hitting the income of private publishing houses and hence attacking private enterprise. It seemed every saving had its cost.

Similar concerns followed the other Rayner scrutinies and the decision to deal with the conflicts they produced by delay appeared to be the policy. It may be that in terms of overall NHS budgets the amounts concerned were small. For example, the implementation of one report on billing insurance companies after treating people involved in road accidents suggested either that the trouble taken to obtain the relatively small sum of £2 million per year was not worth it, or that to make the policy more effective there should be some capital expenditure to provide micro-computers to casualty staff to help them compile the appropriate bills. To many health workers in beleaguered units £2 million would not seem a small amount. The result was no change: the NHS did not want to loose the money, nor invest some to save more. Business efficiency again!

Most of these scrutinies and studies of the organization and practice of the NHS were concentrated on the hospital services. But a firm of consultants, Binder Hamlyn, produced a report commissioned by the DHSS on the family doctor service. The DHSS had a basic problem in that it was not subject to the cash limit policy that, at least, gave a measure of central control in relations with the hospital sector. The government also anticipated a conflict with GPs over deputizing services and was facing a decision on pay rates. Binder Hamlyn's report did not consider it feasible to impose cash limits on GPs but it did suggest other things likely to cause controversy, such as forcing GPs to retire at age 65, restricting medical students entering general practice and restricting the number of foreign doctors coming to the United Kingdom.

General practice was in something of a structural dilemma in that there appeared to be a reduction, overall, in list size for GPs (who were paid on a scale dependent upon numbers registered with them). Suggestions to limit the number of new, rival, GPs or to remove some of the older ones might therefore be welcome. But, at the same time, the direction of government policy was to move towards community care and as such this implied an enhanced role for the GP service. Indeed, the policy was supported by the BMA and assumed a common recognition that it would involve a redistribution of resources from the hospital service to community services (*Guardian*, 4 April 1984). The result was a tentativeness over changes in the GP service typical of a long-running planning dilemma for the NHS. It is assumed that things cannot be fundamentally changed without the consent of the doctors and so they continue their effective veto of the structure of the NHS community services. The stance of the doctors seems to be that if one area of activity is reducing they will gather to themselves others.

As the consultation period for the suggested Griffiths reforms was completed the government decided to appoint 200 general managers to 'run' the NHS. This decision was made despite the continuing levels of criticism from pressure groups and occupational groups, and despite opposition from the House of Commons Social Services Committee. This Committee had submitted detailed criticisms and had not had these answered let alone remedied. The general managers would be phased in over a period of 18 months at regional, district and hospital level (*Guardian*, 7 June 1984).

Of course, the success of the plan depended, in the first instance, on the sorts of people who could fundamentally change the NHS management style being recruited from outside the NHS. Reorganizations in the past had too often meant that people already doing a job had it retitled, carried on doing it and were paid substantially more. Not surprisingly, this reorganization also encountered problems in recruiting the personnel required, or the personnel Griffiths seemed to have in mind to effect changes. Indeed by the end of the year the top job, that of chief executive, the person who would take over national management, had not been filled despite the £60,000 salary being offered.

Potential managers were being offered three-year contracts and 'jobs that offer a real challenge' according to Roy Griffiths. Of the 14 regional health authorities which had appointed general managers 12 had appointed insiders and, by the end of November, at district level, of the 200 appointments made only three were outsiders. One of the three, a British Telecom executive, previously an army colonel, rather unfortunately described his qualifications for the job as including 'an empty mind to look and listen'. But then the Minister of Health, Kenneth Clarke, in trying to make the jobs sound attractive, described the NHS as being 'very complex' and said that 'running the health service was rather like being at the helm of a super tanker in the channel. You can play around with the steering wheel, but the ship just judders a bit and then carries on the way it was going' (*Sunday Times*, 25 November 1984). It was a description that sounded about right but was hardly likely to endear the job to a go-ahead young executive from the private sector contemplating a career move. So one year after the Griffiths Report its major effect seemed to be that a lot of NHS workers were to be paid substantially more, an average of £2000 a year more, to bring the same range of skills to bear on the same problems.

The success of Griffiths was not totally dependent on the recruitment of outside personnel. The proposals also encompassed structural changes and the possibilities for a much closer scrutiny of what was done managerially. Its change in philosophy, a shift from consensus to hierarchical management, would create a different system even with the same personnel. But the problems with recruitment meant a bad start.

While the major focus of interest in terms of structure was centred on the Griffiths reforms, a secondary interest was in the role and composition of health authorities. The Labour Party's health spokesman, Michael Meacher, had commissioned research aimed at identifying what he believed was a growing bias in appointments to health authorities. The 1977 National Health Service Act underlined the authority of the Secretary of State to appoint the 478 regional and district chairmen and regional members. It also identified strict guidelines for the appointment of the 16 members of each district authority. These guidelines said that the ages and sexes should be balanced and that a suitable representation of ethnic minority groups should be encouraged.

Meacher's research results were not clear *vis-à-vis* political bias. But the findings on the composition of authorities indicated that the 1977 Act was far from being implemented. There was not a single person under the age of 25 on any authority; at least 15 people, including chairmen, were aged over 70. Women were outnumbered by men by the proportion of eleven to five. Only two districts had a majority of women. Ethnic minority representation was patchy (*Guardian*, 11 December 1984).

The Labour Party proposed that there be direct elections to health authorities, to be held at the same time as local government polls. Those so elected would replace the appointees of the Secretary of State. As well as introducing a more representative membership, such elections, they argued, would reflect the fact that health authority activity 'is no longer non-political' with authorities discussing things like the closure of facilities and privatization (*Sunday Times*, 16 December 1984). Mr Meacher believed that every chairman but one of a regional health authority was a Conservative and that every local health authority had, in effect, a Conservative majority (*Sunday Times*, 11 November 1984).

The structural preoccupations of 1984 illustrate the problems of innovation in the NHS. The gap between intention and actuality was created and sustained by the coexistence of different interests and understandings. The Labour Party's concern with health authority members seemed somewhat anachronistic in that built into the Griffiths proposals one felt an inexorable shift from members having any effective influence. It was like trying to put right an institutional form destined to ineffectuality anyway. Further, the idea that elections would produce a more representative group on health authorities does not seem to be borne out by the make-up of an elected House of Commons.

During 1985, the continued failure to attract candidates from outside the NHS to general management jobs provoked the DHSS into a more interventionist role. It sought to block, or veto, internal appointments and insisted on outsiders being included on shortlists, if indeed there were any outside applicants. The Minister wanted shortlists both to be approved by him and to be kept secret, in the hope that reluctant businessmen could be attracted (*Guardian*, 8 January 1985). But such setbacks did not stop the moves towards the appointment of unit general managers, the next step in the Griffiths reforms. Indeed some of the new regional and district general managers seemed to want to get very quickly into the reform of a service that still had not really accommodated itself to the structural changes of 1982. The NHS appeared a little like the Football League where when a new manager is appointed he has to sack a player or two, buy in a couple more, change the team's style of play and get results within the first week or two or else he will feel vulnerable to the disfavour of the directors. Indeed three-year contracts were interpreted by some managers as meaning they had to take action quickly in order to be able to show results.

Most of the new management proposals made could be categorized as streamlining, making the management structure more straightforward and more straightforwardly hierarchical. For example, some authorities wanted to abolish the post of chief nursing officer, created in the 1974 Sir Keith Joseph reorganization and redesignated by Mr Fowler in 1982 (*Guardian*, 21 February 1985). Another example of the wish to remove potential countervailing power bases was the suggestion made by 28 district health authorities to drop medical officers from their board of management. These boards of management replaced district management teams and unlike them did not automatically give places to clinicians (*Guardian*, 1 November 1985).

These proposals invoked the wrath of the BMA, which joined with the Royal College of Nursing and protested to the government. This produced an interesting dilemma in the DHSS, a conflict between the new managerialism and the old-fashioned exercise of pressure group power. The latter won and the Minister of Health – by now Barnie Heyhoe had replaced Kenneth Clark – wrote to health authorities saying he 'believed it important that [management] arrangements command the confidence and commitment of all the medical and nursing interests locally' (*Guardian*, 5 December 1985).

The new management structure interacted with entrenched interests and established power bases in the institutions of the NHS (see Halpern 1985). Initial responses varied from the openly confrontational to the surreptitiously undermining or assiduously assimilating. Management was expected to operate in that twilight area between politics and administration. In so doing, it ran the risk of exciting opposition from one or both sides.

Some parallels were being drawn between the Griffiths suggestions and the experience of chief executives in local government. Before 1974 there were a few places with City managers/chief executives but in effect they had no power of direction over other chief officers. In the majority of authorities there was only the chief clerk and these did not appear to assume managerial responsibility. The 1972 Bains Committee made recommendations for reform and chief executives were appointed from 1974. Many of them were the established chief clerks. Since 1974, as new chief executives have been appointed, an initial tendency to appoint lawyers seems to have been replaced with a predominance of accountants. The presence of countervailing power and conflicting interests has been most clearly demonstrated in the struggles between elected councillors and chief executives, with the former fearing the latter would usurp their role as policy-makers and overseers of correct departmental practice. Where councillors have won they have either abolished the post or have added to it specific departmental responsibilities so as to make it too difficult for its holder to do anything by giving him or her too much.

Those relating this local government experience to Griffiths have remarked on the greater degree of central government direction and control in the NHS and the absence of the level of party political practice in its administration (*Health and Social Services Journal*, 3 January 1985, p. 11). These are differences, they suggest, that might facilitate the greater success of general management in the NHS.

Despite setbacks and opposition the new managers seemed to be going about the task of cost cutting with zeal, at least in their dealings with administration. Regional general managers quickly achieved cuts in management costs that, in the main, exceeded the DHSS targets. Only two regions did not. They then proposed another round of savings that would cut 10 per cent of administrative jobs in regional headquarters. The regional general managers felt that this process would be aided by the establishment of national guidelines on good practice. They certainly were conforming to two basic trends, a centralization of power and a preoccupation with the cost, rather than the type or quality, of service.

At the same time as these reforms the health authority audits were being investigated by Michael Meacher, who believed they would reveal a considerable level of abuse of the NHS by consultants involved in private practice (*Guardian*, 11 March 1985). I will look specifically at private practice in a subsequent section but here will note that these revelations were not at odds with a dilemma the DHSS had long recognized – the inability to control the behaviour of the doctors.

At worst doctors could ignore and even undermine the efforts to make services more efficient. For example, doctors in high-profile glamour medicine, such as heart and kidney transplant surgery, have infuriated ministers by launching media campaigns to claim a bigger share of the NHS budget. The heart unit at Guy's Hospital, London, for example, appeared to be deliberately overspending its budget. Kenneth Clark, as Minister of Health, said of this: 'If they use public uproar as an alternative to cooperating with the management we will have to get them to realise that they will get nowhere. In the last resort the place will shut' (*Sunday Times*, 17 March 1985). Guy's was breaking the rules even in the pressure group politics of the NHS where one of the prices the doctors pay for the considerable influence of the BMA is a requirement to act along the channels it has set up and exploits so well. If they break the rules then much else is thrown into the melting pot. For example, the DHSS will use the power of audit to follow up the exploitation of the NHS by doctors with private patients (referring one doctor to the Director of Public Prosecutions for fraud) and they made oblique references to the possibility of scrapping jobs-for-life contracts for consultants.

If the dominant issue presented by Griffiths was what sort of management structure the NHS should have, the issue in the implementation of Griffiths was who should manage. The new structure in the DHSS, the Management Board, and the tighter controls over money that the reforms would herald, were designed to underline the reality that it was the DHSS who allocated resources and set priorities and not the doctors. There was to be a new approach based on accountability, both for results achieved and for resources used and costs incurred (Nickson 1985, p. 41), and on efficiency. The specificity of the economic measurement as opposed to the difficulty of measuring outcome was one factor that was increasingly likely to transform this concept into a more purely economic mode. Indeed, efficiency was to be measured even more explicitly in terms of resources used.

The triumph of managerialism was a reality not universally accepted, either structurally or conceptually. Consultants still held the exclusive right to admit and discharge from hospital and they were certain that this was not something they would give up to non-medical general managers. Consultants' leader, Paddy Ross, speaking on BBC Radio 4 *File on Four* just after the Annual Conference of Consultants in 1985, summed up the understanding of the nature of the NHS that they now wished to be associated with like this:

> The concept of the NHS was to provide an administrative system within which doctors treated patients in the light of their professional judgement. The NHS is just the system that pays the bills and provides the hospitals and all that. Doctors see their prime allegiance to the patient and not to the system.

Another debate that addresses related issues was joined in 1985. Professor Williams (1985) presented the notion of the Quality Adjusted Life Year (QALY) with the aim of introducing individual preferences in such a way as to allow them to be used to assess rationally the benefits of alternative treatments. The cost effectiveness of different treatments could be calculated and this would add the voice of a constituency wider than the medical profession in making decisions about resource allocation. Williams was correctly pointing out that priorities always have to be set and there is a clear case for doing this in a more open way, not leaving it to the providers of the service to make decisions for the potential users. The debate achieved more than an academic interest because it was widely taken up in those journals, such as *HSSJ*, much read by NHS workers, and because it coincided with publicity being given to a decision of Oxford Health Authority to decline to provide further kidney dialysis for Mr Derek Sage, a patient in its care.

When money is short not everyone can get all they need and traditionally the decision of who gets what had been taken in such a way that responsibility could not be clearly located and hence the rationale of that choice not questioned. Further, there exists the inclination to respond first to more dramatic needs where medicine can be seen to be 'doing something', the perennial determinate for much resource allocation. Professor Williams confronts us with this by posing the dilemma of how we explain to 'several crippled and housebound old ladies in a lot of pain that they cannot have [hip replacement] operations because we've decided a fifty five year old man who gets chest pain when he over exerts himself should have priority' (*Guardian*, 27 February 1985).

Professor Williams was addressing a fundamental change in the true nature of medicine that may not be widely appreciated in allocation policies. At an earlier point in its development medicine was primarily about infectious disease. New treatments could be shown to be effective in the impact they had on mortality. Even here, as was demonstrated in McKeown's (1979) work, the nature of causal relationships was not always understood. But now much medicine is concerned with the response to chronic and degenerative conditions, and for many patients the concept of cure does not come into the question. The problem is how to assess the resources that should be located in this sort of treatment as opposed to the more overtly cure-based. He is also writing at a time when there is a struggle between management and clinical power and, in a sense, he is adding another voice to this. He calls it the voice of the potential consumer and the eventual payer but it does sound like the voice of the academic and researcher. Williams schema claims to add the rational voice to the responsible voice of the administrator and the professional voice of the clinician.

The one other factor that seemed significant in terms of NHS structure in 1985 was an ongoing dispute about the size of the NHS drugs bill and what measures could be taken to reduce it. In November 1984 Norman Fowler had issued a restricted list of drugs that could be prescribed. It was expected that this would save £160 million at virtually no political cost. It did mean taking on the doctors about the freedom to prescribe, and sure enough the BMA had objected. What emerged in early 1985 was the realization that even for those who might support the principle of such a list the way it had been presented and the details of the list would not just reduce the choice of the doctor in terms of the way a patient is treated but would in fact prevent some people being treated at all (Le Fanu 1985). It was a report from the Standard Medical Advisory Committee (which includes representatives of the Royal Colleges) which pointed this out and the plans were modified. In effect, this modification amounted to an increase in the number of drugs permitted to be prescribed and a corresponding reduction in the savings the whole exercise would produce (*Guardian*, 22 February 1985). It showed the Minister as being badly briefed and left him embarrassed over a scheme he had hoped would be relatively uncontentious. Losing a round of a long fight on points makes it harder to recover the ground in the next one.

The issue of the restricted list highlighted some of the conflicts in ideology evident within both the Conservative and Labour Parties. Conservatives may have wished to control public expenditure but, certainly from the back-benches in Parliament, there were arguments that a restricted list would be unfairly discriminatory against certain products of certain drug companies and that it would interfere with free choice on the part of the doctor and of the patient. Here in microcosm are the conflicts continually evident in a Conservative Party trying to reconcile the irreconcilable. Labour was divided, happy to see the drug companies taken on but apprehensive that the measures proposed would encourage private medicine. Further, the scheme would be prejudicial to the interests of the old and the chronic sick. According to Labour's health spokesman, Frank Dobson, they would suffer because 'it is no good telling an old person they can no longer have the cough mixture they have used for years'. He feared that person would have to buy it on the open market. Other Labour supporters, though, saw the list as a useful device to make doctors prescribe more carefully, to reduce the influence of dubious advertising and to curb the excesses of the multinational drug companies (*Sunday Times*, 17 March 1985).

The problems identified with the drafting of the Bill were that the list was criticized as too narrow. Certain patients would need specific named drugs and these would not be available. The impact might be to push prescribing up towards more potent substances. Doctors unable to prescribe a now restricted tonic may choose to suggest, and prescribe, a non-restricted more powerful drug. Such objections led to compromise and a shift from the letter and the spirit of the proposed change. First, the list of approved drugs was expanded. Then doctors were given permission to prescribe restricted drugs and argue their case at a medical committee later. The drug companies spent £1 million campaigning against the list but one senses that it was a battle that could have been won by the government with a little more effective drafting and tactics.

1986 began with a series of full-page advertisements in national newspapers issued by the Royal College of Nursing. These contained criticism of the Griffiths changes and their impact on nursing, calling attention to 'the most radical change in the structure of Britain's health care ever' which would exclude nurses from any management decisions at all. They were making a case for the recognition of the particular contribution of nursing with its commitment and expertise. Nurses should run nursing and there should be a director of nursing in every hospital, clinic and health unit. These directors should work with the administrator. They identified nursing with the caring component in health care and called the nurse the patient's spokesman. The campaign cost £250,000.

In March the government announced that it was not reappointing 62 of the 170 district health authority chairmen. This followed a vetting process carried out by Conservative Central Office which was designed to identify those chairmen who had fought the government's cuts in the NHS. It was those so identified that, disproportionately, did not get reappointed even if they were generally identified as Conservative supporters (*Guardian*, 13 March 1986; 19 March 1986).

By April enough new-style managers were in post to get some sense of where they came from and what attitudes they might bring to the NHS. Thirteen health authorities appointed former military officers, presumably for their 'leadership qualities'. Others came from the commercial world. One merchandising director of an Oxford Street store took over as general manager for the John Radcliffe Hospital, Oxford.

At the Management Board level the new Chairman, Victor Paige, had previously been at the Port of London Authority. The Director of Personnel, Len Peach, had previously been Director of Personnel and Corporate Affairs at IBM. The Director of Financial Management, Ian Mills, had been a senior partner in management consultants, Price Waterhouse. But despite these 'successes' still only 10 per cent of the new posts were filled by people from outside the NHS.

However, the role of the private sector was enhanced by an increasing recourse to employing private management consultants. Spending by the DHSS on management consultants had gone up from £411,000 in 1979 to £13.8 million in 1985. Phil Cohen (1986) called this whole process 'privatisation from within', a way of making the NHS lucrative for the private sector and a way of introducing a management structure that would be more amenable and more able to carry through the government's plans. The market for such management consultancy was far from exhausted, with many districts still not getting involved. Other forms of privatization, although making a significant impact, were still not dominant. For example, in the provision of ancillary services by the end of 1985 private contractors had won 107 tenders with 258 staying with direct-labour NHS teams. Fourteen thousand ancillary workers had been lost from the NHS in 1985 due to privatization.

Another person soon lost was Victor Paige, who resigned in June. Did he jump or was he pushed? Did he press for too many cuts or too few? These were the questions the Opposition put to Mr Fowler in the Commons when the news became known. It did appear that a series of disputes had developed between Paige and Fowler. One interpretation of these was that Paige went about doing what he thought he had been appointed to do and managed in the new style. But he did not appreciate the political dimension that Mr Fowler had to consider. For example, Paige was reputed to wish to press on with the sale of nurses' homes, whereas Mr Fowler expressed some reservations about evicting nurses. Paige wanted to establish a rational pay structure for new general managers in which where you came from would have a major impact on the salary you were offered, while Fowler wanted to delay this. The Secretary of State also delayed the announcement of the decisions on which health authority chairmen would be replaced. It appeared that Mr Paige sought and did not get clarity. Some attribute this to Mr Fowler's reluctance to take decisions he could be criticized for, others to the problems the new ministers Hayhoe and Whitney had setting priorities, and still others to the subtle undermining of Mr Paige's position by established Civil Servants whose interests were not served by this appointment being successful (*Guardian*, 5 June 1986).

In announcing Mr Paige's departure to the House of Commons, Mr Fowler was quick to locate it in the context of what he saw as the overall success of the scheme of appointing general managers. Seven hundred and fifty had been appointed, he said, and only two or three had left. There certainly seemed an inevitability about the conflict between a Griffiths-style manager and the considerations of political expediency. Equally inevitable was the clash with the established bureaucratic machinery. What was not inevitable was that it should be concluded with the very public resignation of the manager.

In drawing up guidelines for the appointment of a replacement some of the true nature of this conflict was apparent. The new person appointed would have to take a public share of the responsibility for the consequences of unpopular decisions (presumably the Minister would be able to manage to give the good news himself). The plan was that after important policy decisions the new appointee would appear on TV and radio and give newspaper interviews so as to 'draw political fire away from the Government and individual ministers' (*Guardian*, 16 June 1986).

At about the same time an interesting interview appeared with the Director of Personnel, Len Peach (*Guardian*, 9 June 1986). He was reported as being slightly shell-shocked at the amount of public attention given to NHS management and said that work at the NHS was like work in a goldfish bowl. He described the setting as having a very democratic basis with debates in public. Those of us who have spent time studying the DHSS and bureaucracy in general may find this description surprising. Perhaps we should appreciate just how secretive and hierarchical the idealized private sector is. Peach described the Griffiths Report as 'his Bible' and in order to implement it he argued for the need to appoint managers who were personally accountable and whose performance could be reviewed and evaluated. Additionally he supported the introduction of performance-related pay. As to the conflict between management and the political requirements of the Secretary of State, he sidestepped that with the familiar formula of separate spheres – strategy as the preserve of the politician and management decisions for the managers. It was a formula that clearly had not worked for Victor Paige.

The Labour Party, at this time, seemed to have accepted the reality of the Griffiths reforms and decided that it would not introduce another management change should it have the opportunity. It argued that the worst thing for the NHS would be yet another upheaval (even worse than continuing with general management). But it would want to reinforce the accountability of general managers to elected district health authorities, in the way that chief executives were accountable to elected local authorities. Michael Meacher also criticized the kinds of people appointed to the general manager posts: 'Patients don't want their health service run by a brigadier or the manager of a food chain, but by people with experience, dedication and feel for the NHS' (*Guardian*, 27 June 1986).

In September the DHSS announced the introduction of a merit pay system for general managers and unit managers. It was described by the health trade unions as an incentive scheme for accelerating hospital closures and service cuts. In fact the criteria for pay increases were very closely linked to local factors like performance in reducing unit costs, reductions in waiting lists and maintaining financial controls. The means for assessment was that health authority chairmen would conduct the review of their own managers with a referral up to the next level for approval. Although it was expected that some managers would receive an extra 20 per cent through this scheme, the procedure of upward referral would ensure that not everyone received the top payment (*Guardian*, 4 September 1986). Such variations in payment, it was generally assumed, would enhance the degree to which NHS activity could be controlled from the centre. This would make it consistent with the overall direction of change and further highlight the contradiction between the rhetoric of encouraging local initiative and independent enterprise and the reality of an enhanced system of scrutiny and now reward to ensure the compliance of region, district and units with central direction.

The tendency towards centralization was enhanced in October when the Health Minister, Tony Newton, was appointed to chair the Management Board. He replaced Victor Paige, with the temporary chairman, Len Peach, being made Chief Executive to the Board. Sir Roy Griffiths became part-time Deputy Chairman and had direct access, as government adviser on NHS management, to the Prime Minister. The change was presented as one designed to integrate managers and ministers and so give a clear central line of communication. Norman Fowler, in presenting the change, sought to clarify that there was no way in which the Board could be independent of the Minister because the NHS was directly funded and ministers were responsible to Parliament for it. He put it thus: 'The Management Board is to see that things get done ... the Health Service is a complex organisation and ministers could not run everything' (*Guardian*, 3 October 1986). The Board would stay within the DHSS but would give leadership to health authorities, would monitor performance and ensure effective use of resources. In addition to the Management Board there would be a Supervisory Board, meeting less frequently and chaired by the Secretary of State. This would include other departmental ministers, the DHSS Permanent Secretary and the chief medical and nursing officers.

That this was a shift towards centralization seemed to be underlined by the discussion at a conference for the 14 regional managers in October. The discussion centred on future trends and the assumption appeared to be that there would be 'profound management changes over the next five years'. The direction of these changes was to create a national health service rather than what had been a 35-year-old loose federation. At least this was the sense of the meeting as summarized by one of the managers present, John Hoare of Wessex, in a confidential memorandum subsequently reported in the *Guardian* (29 December 1986), as is the way with confidential memoranda. He identified two main factors prompting this centralization, the belief that the devolved health service had failed to deliver in a number of areas, and the pressure from the House of Commons Public Accounts Committee underlining the constitutional point that ministers are responsible for the implementation of policy. He identified the struggle between Victor Paige and Norman Fowler as being important and its resolution with the departure of Paige and the appointment of the Health Minister to chair the Management Committee as being a notable victory for the politicians. What would be important to review was whether the Management Board now had any authority independent of the Supervisory Board.

The leaked memorandum also referred to the directives from ministers on privatizing catering and cleaning and other economy measures. This is identified with a diminution of the scope of district health authorities to make decisions about even operational matters. What is being eroded is the scope for local discretion, which appeared intrinsic to the whole idea of management initiatives to adapt a service to meet local needs and resources.

If these changes are identified with the wish to give the NHS a corporate identity this will have serious implications for the role of regions and districts and even more so for the members of authorities at each of these levels. The system, as it was evolving, had built into it an important role for health authority chairmen, not least in the arrangements for deciding merit bonuses. But the role of the member was increasingly difficult to identify.

Other issues related to structure during the year included the pre-election manoeuvring of the Labour Party to address some of the issues of management and accountability. Areas discussed included the relationship between health authorities and local authorities and the possible changes that could encourage a greater degree of democratic accountability in health. It was an interesting repeat of the discussions in the Crossman/Keith Joseph years in which the Labour Party adopted the position that it was the kind of service and its structure of control that were important and the Conservatives looked to performance and value for money (*Guardian*, 2 August 1986; 29 October 1986; see also Ham 1985). This sort of development was related to the GP services, with Labour considering the establishment of annual meetings for patients of family doctors (*Observer*, 7 September 1986).

In 1987 the amount of public debate over the Griffiths reforms decreased notably. It was to be an election year and the issues of spending and cutbacks seemed to dominate. Cost and performance not organization preoccupied commentators. Indeed the central issue concerning structure appeared to be the place of health education. When such fringe activities occupy centre stage it must be indicative of an absence of news and development from the real concerns of the NHS!

In November 1986, ostensibly as part of the development of a strategic response to the health problems of AIDS, Norman Fowler announced his intention to dissolve the Health Education Council (HEC) and reconstitute it as a health authority, the Health Education Authority (HEA). The new authority would be responsible for running the AIDS programme, with its £20 million funding. This change produced mixed responses. It could be construed as bringing health education more nearly into the centre of health planning and as such enhancing its status. Or it could be seen as a device that would enable the DHSS to control the work of the authority and prevent the production of reports embarrassing to the government. Was this just another manifestation of the move towards centralization? Dr David Player, Director of the Health Education Council, certainly felt that its abolition would achieve greater governmental control and in so doing reassure the pressure group interests that the HEC had antagonized, specifically the tobacco and alcohol industries (*Guardian*, 13 February 1987).

In a move reminiscent of the *Yes, Prime Minister* episode where an MP spokesman for the tobacco industry was made Minister of Health, a director of a market research firm with clients in the alcohol and tobacco industries was appointed Vice-Chairman of the new authority. Ann Burdus had worked for a firm which had the distinction of making the eighth biggest donation to the Conservative Party from a company, £50,000, in 1983. She did not think there would be a problem. The new health authority's first job was to launch a campaign against heart disease in which people would be advised to stop smoking and switch from dairy fats. Mrs Burdus's company had as clients Embassy cigarettes and the dairy industry (*Guardian*, 19 February 1987). One of the company's associate directors who was commisioned to work on health authority contracts asked to have 'National No Smoking Day' off as working it might involve her in a conflict of interests (*Guardian*, 20 February 1987)!

David Player had been suspicious about the role of pressure groups in the demise of the HEC. But perhaps even more pervasive was the sense of the government wanting to avoid exposés on the failings of health provision in general. The HEC had commissioned a report to update the Black Report (Townsend and Davidson 1982) on inequalities in health. The report highlighted the health gap between rich and poor and indicated that it had become wider under the Conservatives (Health Education Council 1987). It did appear that the new authority, and its Chairman, Sir Brian Bailey, after advice from the DHSS, engaged in a crude attempt to block its publication. This certainly led to doubts about the degree of independence the new body would show (*Guardian*, 26 March 1987). The circumstances around the eventual publication of the report bordered on farce. They were followed by the appointment of a new manager for the authority, Dr Spencer Hagard, who started work on April Fool's Day. (Dr David Player did not get the job!)

The HEC always existed with uncertainty as to its budget and its staffing. As a quango it could be easily abolished (Sutherland 1987). But it had pursued a line that risked taking on the powerful pressure groups and confronting the relationship between poverty and ill health. In 1987 it was hard to envisage the new authority doing the same.

A more ongoing area of concern emerged in a report issued in April in which the House of Commons Committee of Public Accounts (1987) questioned the real control the House was having, or could have, over government expenditure. Whitehall departmental estimates are vague and the connection between the Treasury's Expenditure White Paper and the Supply Estimates is far from clear. Even where there is sufficient detail this is not located in the context of objectives and targets for which the spending is designed. Thus Parliament's ability to have any effective scrutiny is undermined.

Paradoxically this complaint is at odds with, in health, a shift towards a closer scrutiny of spending and performance. It is as if Whitehall is heading in the opposite direction to the rules it is seeking to impose upon the health regions and districts. This is, in reality, a further example of the exercise of executive power. It is not so much that information is not provided. The Treasury provides five documents a year for Parliament, the Financial Statement and Budget Report; the Autumn Statement (published normally in November); the Public Expenditure White Paper (published in January); the Supply Estimates (sent to the Commons in March); and the Appropriation Accounts (published in the Autumn following the end of the financial year). It is, rather, the form in which information is made available. To be effective information needs to be presented in a way that optimises the opportunity for MPs to use it and not in a way that mystifies and confuses (House of Commons Committee of Public Accounts 1987).

In 1987 pilot studies were set up in hospitals in three health districts – Newcastle, the Wirral and Huddersfield – in which information would be provided to doctors and nurses about the costs of what they did with patients. This utilized an American technique of classifying hospital treatments by diagnosis and measuring the resources used (in what were to be known as Diagnosis Related Groups (DRGs)). The government explained the pilot project as being something that would enable the cost, efficiency and quality of health care to be evaluated. This would facilitate a concentration of resources in areas that do best. For example, if one hospital appears particularly good (on these criteria) at a certain sort of treatment then patients from other hospitals might be transferred to it (*Independent*, 21 April 1987). Such ideas became linked with a discussion about the internal market in the NHS, of which more later.

The year saw the continuation of the now regular disputes between doctors and administrators. One consultant, in April, struck a resonant note when he complained about the absence of any professional code of conduct for managers. Hence there was an absence of redress or censure of their actions in so far as they conform to, or confound, a professional standard. He argued that managers were increasingly deciding the nature of patient care, for example by allocating nursing levels to specific wards. Such management decisions could be detrimental to patients but managers and administrators had neither a code of conduct nor an independent disciplinary body to which complaints of misconduct could be made (R.F. Heys, writing to the *Guardian*, 10 April 1987).

This was not to say that the managers did not have a collective voice. In May the Institute of Health Service Management, in evidence to the House of Commons Social Services Committee, said that the NHS was one of the most undermanaged public services in any of the industrialized countries. Its advice to the Commons was that investing more money in management would be cost effective in helping patient care. Figures in support of this advice identified a cut in support staff by 21,000 between 1978 and 1985, while direct care staff, such as nurses and doctors, increased by 72,000. The veracity of these figures should not be assumed or at least not accepted as uncontested. It is also the case that there is not necessarily a direct relationship between the numbers of support staff and their influence. It's not just who they are but what structural position they are in (*Guardian*, 26 May 1987)!

An emphasis on cost control created the anxiety that a health district would not want to treat someone else's patients. Cross-boundary patient flows in such an environment become a major cause of concern. Such problems were identified in a National Association of Health Authorities (1987) report. Districts were refusing to take patients from other districts unless the latter agreed to pay. A story often repeated by those eager to criticize private enterprise health schemes concerns the United States. Its scenario is of a potential patient being shifted from one hospital to another because it was not clear that the patient could pay, until one was found that would take a chance or until the patient died. The concerns about cross-boundary flow provoked similar anxieties in the United Kingdom.

Such concerns are evident because of a tendency within the NHS for specialisms to develop within particular hospitals. A utilization of DRGs would further promote such a trend. General practitioners could refer patients to the hospital they considered most appropriate and that might be within another district. The existing situation was that one district did pay another but it was generally agreed that the cost charged was not the true cost, was often paid up to two years late and the system worked to the detriment of some districts.

Centralizing control did not change the experienced reality that it was the service deliverers in units at district level that were seen as having to make the face-to-face rationing decisions. If the government's message was of unprecedented spending and the local experience was of shortage, of a decline in facilities (number and standard) and of low morale then who was the patient to blame? In a speech to the Institute of Health Service Management in June that organization's president said that rationing issues had been effectively

> dumped on doctors, nurses, receptionists and porters. They had to tell patients why conditions were unsatisfactory, or why some sorts of treatment were not available. It surfaced in public health authority meetings when rational choices on priority presented by district managers appeared to the public as undeniable unmet demands (Barbara Young, quoted in the *Guardian*, 11 June 1987).

The writer was arguing for a more public acknowledgment of the 'resource collision' at regional and local levels and also for a planning system that acknowledged the future difficulties to be faced and did not base plans on 'acts of faith'.

Other issues current in 1987 included continuing examination of the role of drug companies and an ongoing debate about GPs and their susceptibility to the new managerialism. Nursing also figured as an area of concern, in part because of what was perceived as a demographic problem related to the dwindling number of school leavers. Nursing regularly draws on a section of the female school-leaving cohort who have obtained between 5 O levels and one A level, recruiting 25 per cent of this group in the mid 1980s. But this cohort was decreasing in number at a time when it was likely that there would be an increase in the need for nurses because of the rising age of the population as a whole. Nursing would need to attract almost 50 per cent of its usual target group by the year 1995 to maintain the service required (*Guardian*, 24 March 1987). The NHS is beset by demographic problems!

Of course, this problem remains only if nursing retains its established career structure and recruitment policy. One change the UK Central Council for Nursing, Midwifery and Health Visiting contemplated was the recruitment of more men, another was to upgrade recruitment and the form of training, to expect and consequently also be able to offer more to nurses. The Royal College of Nursing has gone further and suggested that nurse training should shift into higher education. It is to the profession's credit that at a time when education was under attack it should emphasize the value of extra academic study.

Nursing has always suffered from problems of retaining the staff its recruits. Isobel Menzies (1960) presented a most influential analysis of why this should be. Thirty-five per cent of trainee nurses either fail or leave their course. One problem inhibiting recruitment and influential in established nurses leaving the profession is the low pay. Without large proportions of low-paid workers the NHS financial position would be even more serious than it is. For example, according to DHSS figures, 46 per cent of nursing staff caring for geriatric and mentally handicapped patients are nursing auxiliaries and a further 11 per cent of those dealing with the mentally handicapped are students or pupils. These grades are required to carry out jobs, such as the administration of drugs and the supervision of wards, that are neither included in their training nor recognized in their pay (Rahman 1987).

The then current rate of 30,000 nurses a year leaving the profession was brought to Mrs Thatcher's attention in Parliament on 7 April 1987. She summarized her understanding of the present position of nurses as being that they now worked a reduced number of hours a week, the total number employed had gone up and they received pay that was one-third higher in real terms than in 1979, without the value of their last pay increase being included.

The disparity between an apparent statistical reality presented by the Prime Minister and an expressed, or acted-out, felt reality evident in the feelings of nurses and in their rate of departure from the profession is indicative of a fundamental paradox of communication about the NHS in the 1980s.

5   Public Expenditure and Cuts in the National Health Service

Of course, the very title of this chapter is contentious and, as I offer it, suggests that some conclusion about the nature of policy-making in health has already been drawn. I will try and present the evidence and will begin with the impressions of the immediate and likely impact of the changes in funding announced in July 1983 by the Chancellor and changes in staffing announced by Norman Fowler, the Secretary of State, in September of that year. If in my chapter on structure it was the Griffiths Report (DHSS 1983a) that marked a starting point, then a convenient one in terms of cuts or changes in services are these funding announcements.

The 1983 summer and autumn changes amounted to a cut of £80 million and job losses of 5000 in the NHS. A survey published in January 1984 (*Guardian*, 18 January 1984) reported the results of a questionnaire sent to all 199 district health authorities in England and Wales. Seventy-two authorities had replied (in itself that might be a reply rate that invalidates some of the findings because it may have been self-selecting, with replies coming only from those in sympathy with the imputed intentions of the questionnaire). Nevertheless, it did provide data not available elsewhere. The DHSS, under Patrick Jenkin, had decided to abolish that division which supplied much of the information available to ministers. The consequence was that the data available both to make decisions and to follow up their consequences became much more limited and, because data would be recorded in different ways in future, historical analysis would become more difficult. The survey also indicates major areas of concern within, at least, the 36 per cent of districts which had replied.

Some of the effects of cuts had been almost immediate, others seemed to be setting up problems for the future. In the latter case the survey identified a trend to economize by postponing improvements in the generally targeted priority areas such as the mentally ill, handicapped and elderly. A group of 21 health authorities, with South-East England and London over-represented, reported that the cuts had necessitated the closure of hospitals, wards or clinics. Another group identified the major impact as being not closure but the halting of plans for expansion (generally authorities in East Anglia, the South-West and the North). These authorities included those, like Norwich, which reported that they did not have to cut but could only maintain what they identified as a service that was already not meeting the needs of patients, and those, like West Norfolk, where a service did not come up to the DHSS's own targets and would now stand no chance of improving towards these.

One problem created by dividing the cuts exercise between financial controls and staffing limits was that it became possible, and in a number of cases was indeed evident, that authorities under-spending at the time of the cuts might still be under-spending but were not allowed to increase their staffing complement despite their being able to 'afford' it according to the government's criteria.

The staffing exercise was widely criticized. Tunbridge Wells District Health Authority's administrator called it 'crude, indiscriminate, and irrational, creating a tremendous workload and bad press for little overall effect'. Plymouth's administrator commented on the broader impact of the whole exercise when he described the imposed changes as making 'absolute nonsense of planning. If plans are changed at short notice it invariably means a complete waste of time and money' (Guardian, 18 January 1984).

The debate continued to centre on two main themes. The first was an identification of specific cuts and the impact they were having. The second was the debate about levels of spending and the claim that never before had so much been spent. Typical stories from the first half of January 1984 illustrate this schizoid discourse. Doctors at Wythenshawe Hospital in Manchester reported that patients were dying because of a shortage of nurses and beds. Six patients waiting for heart surgery had died within four weeks of Christmas and those deaths had been preventable. The health authority responded by saying that the number of heart operations performed had increased and more operations were carried out than had been budgeted for. But the need continued to grow faster than the provision, not so much because of an increase in the number of sufferers but because of rates of referral to this well-known resource. Further, the health authority had to balance claims for funding heart surgery with the need for more kidney dialysis and more cancer treatment (Guardian, 6 January 1984).

A few days after these specific examples had appeared in the Press the Secretary of State was publicizing an increase in spending £83 million to 'restore the previous July's cuts and to slightly increase spending overall'. He foresaw, with further savings in manpower and costs, that even more could be diverted in patient care. This might be translated as another manifestation of the workers paying for the NHS and is based on calculating wage increases at a rate below inflation, 3 per cent rather than 5 per cent. It is an invidious process saying that if you have more heart operations kidney patients will die and even more so to say that health workers must become poorer to help the NHS break even or grow (*Guardian*, 11 January 1984). More than one-third of adult full-time male workers and three-quarters of adult female full-time workers covered by the Ancillary Staffs Council in the NHS earn less than two-thirds of national average earnings. Catering and laundry staff fall below the statutory minimum laid down by wages councils and cleaners earn less than the average for cleaners in industry. To restore the position current in 1975 when a £30 a week minimum – then equivalent to two-thirds of average wages – was in force would, in 1984, have required a 22.1 per cent increase and not the 3 per cent being offered (*Guardian*, 6 March 1984).

By April confusion was widespread. An Office of Health Economics (OHE) survey revealed that spending on the NHS would reach a record £17 billion in 1984, figures which they said represented a growth in real terms of 1 per cent a year for the last three years. But this was a figure that did not take into account the higher costs of equipment and drugs (the OHE is the drug industries research unit). The NHS in 1984 absorbed 6.2 per cent of Gross National Product as opposed to 6.1 per cent in 1981 (Office of Health Economics 1984). At the same time the Press were reporting that the NHS appeared to have suffered spending cuts of nearly £130 million and lost more than 8000 jobs, figures even in excess of the targets set by Norman Fowler in 1983. Many health authorities reported that they had under-spent. Oxford Regional Health Authority, for example, experienced cuts of £2.6 million and in addition under-spent by a further £425,000 (*Guardian*, 6 April 1984). They were neither alone nor the most severely under-spent. Planning was consequently in a state of considerable confusion.

Staying with this confusion, in March the Medical Research Council announced that it would cut funds to its 56 units by £3 million in 1984. Directors of these units had been warned that such cuts would severely affect research into causes and cures of disease. They amounted to actual cuts in the recurring costs of research of 16 per cent with no allowance for inflation, an effective further cut of 5 per cent. Later in the year as these cuts began to work through to field centres it meant that, for example, a research team at Addenbrooke's Hospital in Cambridge researching cot deaths was closed down. Cot deaths are the most frequent cause of infant mortality after the first week of life, with 1200 deaths a year in England and Wales (*Guardian*, 28 June 1984).

Shortly after these research cuts were announced the annual merit awards to consultants were made public. They totalled £42 million. Merit awards are best understood as the continuation of the 'stuffing mouths with gold' that is supposed to have tied the allegiance of consultants to the

NHS. (By the mid-1980s the proportion who now worked part-time and supplemented their income from private practice was so great that use of the term 'allegiance' can appear opportunistic rather than descriptive.) Merit awards are recommended by a medical advisory panel whose deliberations are secret. The distribution of the awards by discipline, by geography and by gender appears far from fair. The awards are most often made to those in high-status, high-technology specialisms. They are much more often received by men and are disproportionately distributed in favour of the South-East. Awards are given to 58.6 per cent of specialists in cardio-thoracic medicine and to only 24.2 per cent of community physicians. In 1982 only 15 per cent of female consultants got awards as opposed to 37.9 per cent of male. Of these, only one woman in England and Wales got the top award while 119 men did. (In 1984 there was a 100 per cent increase in the number of women getting the top award – to two.) A research report on this phenomenon in the *British Medical Journal* (reported in the *Guardian*, 23 May 1984) concluded that 'we are observing the universal tendency for self regarding groups to allocate prizes to people as much like themselves as possible'.

These awards are difficult to reconcile with the financial shortages prevalent in the NHS; as some critics of the system said to the *Guardian*'s reporter, 'the money could be better spent on essential services'. They also reinforce a hierarchy within the profession that is not only discriminatory but does not correspond to the contemporary needs of a health service in 1980s Britain. The sums involved for individuals are considerable – the top award is of £20,825! (By 1988 that sum had increased to £33,720.) Merit awards are supported by consultants' organizations not just for the obvious reasons but because, it is argued, a flat rate for all consultants would – if politicians were so inclined – make the imposition of an entire flat rate service easier.

In June the government, in effect, cut the planned growth of 1 per cent in the NHS by a half in that they approved pay rises for doctors and nurses without fully funding them. The increases amounted to between 6 and 8 per cent for nurses and 4 and 6 per cent for doctors and dentists. This added £216 million to the NHS budget on top of the 3 per cent the government had already calculated for pay increases. Of that £180 million would come from the contingency reserve but health authorities would have to find the other £36 million from the £85 million growth money allowed in the year's budget and from savings they had planned (*The Times*, 8 June 1984).

Ancillary workers, technicians, craftsmen and white-collar staff had been offered 3 per cent in this same package. These workers had been split off from the nurses in regard to decisions over pay by the introduction of a review body for nurses' pay. The intention of this new procedure was to separate the politically sensitive decisions over nurses pay from the group *The Times* (28 June 1984) editorial writer called 'the large low paid but less overworked and less sympathised with category of NHS ancillary workers'.

If we link these decisions over finance with those concurrently affecting structural change we see the considerable problem of developing either a coherent planning strategy or even a management programme with any medium- or long-term perspective when the resources available can be so drastically changed.

The annual report on the NHS DHSS (1984a) clarified some of the issues about the reality of spending figures in the NHS. But sufficient detail was obscure, or disputed, and the picture remained complex. Over the past five years, the report said, spending on health care had doubled in cash terms. But in real terms it had only grown by 7 per cent when the increased costs to the NHS, above inflation rates, were taken into account. The Secretary of State had claimed a 17 per cent increase above the retail price index, but this index did not include many of the items the NHS required. These had risen significantly faster. The factor not included in either of these figures was the increased demand consequent upon changes in population structure. In 1984 there were more admissions and out-patient appointments than ever before. But then the means of calculating these and the impact of the practice of early discharge and consequent higher readmission rates meant that the actual number treated, as opposed to the number of treatments, was not among the figures presented to Parliament.

In all health districts this national scenario was having implication for local planning and practice. In Bradford District Health Authority, for example, attention was concentrated on the fate of two hospitals, Shipley and Thornton View. Both were for the elderly and the authority argued that the district was over-supplied with beds in this particular specialism. If both hospitals were closed then a resulting saving of over £1 million a year could be used to help rebuild a major local general hospital, St Lukes. There were campaigns to save both threatened hospitals. Thornton View's centred on an occupation and received widespread support from trade unionists, Labour Party politicians, local health professionals and relatives of people in, or previously at, the hospital. Shipley was in the constituency of Conservative MP Marcus Fox, who warned the government of a widespread grassroots revolt (even evident in the local Conservative Party) which would jeopardize his seat if Shipley Hospital were closed (Cohen 1984b). The end result of the campaigns was that Thornton View was closed and Shipley was subject to a change of use and remained open. The campaigns concerned with the closure of these hospitals illustrated the continuing dominance of short-term political considerations over management independence and financial judgement and highlighted the impact of opposition within the dominant structure as opposed to that expressed outside it.

Even if the government accepted the argument that the NHS had to grow by nearly 2 per cent per year just to keep pace with demographic and technological changes, this did not imply a commitment or even an intention to increase expenditure commensurately. The Health Minister, Barney Heyhoe, speaking in January 1985, made the picture clear when he spoke of the need for greater efficiency and low wage settlements. The government would not, he said, pick up the bill for pay settlements above the previously budgeted percentage. He continued:

> Health Authorities cannot expect, any more than employers in other industries and services, to be insulated from uncertainty over the level of pay settlements, and it would be wholly unrealistic to expect the Exchequer to pick up whatever costs arose (*Guardian*, 30 January 1985).

This was one of those ministerial statements that attempts to create what it exhorts. To claim that something is self-evidently what all right-thinking people must accept is 'Emperor's new clothes' logic. It does not stand critical examination. For example, we might ask why health authorities, which do not participate in the actual negotiations that determine the pay settlement they then have to implement, should be treated in the same way as other concerns which do participate.

The NHS Management Board was encouraging health authorities to sell off land surplus to their requirements. These sales might go some way towards allowing them, with their limited allocations of money, to make a one-off contribution to funds that could be used for growth. The closure of hospitals presented the opportunity for land sales, as did the disposal of the extensive grounds around some hospitals. The hospital would remain open though with much nearer neighbours! It was a proposal criticized as akin to selling of the family silver to pay the grocer's bill. But such asset stripping was consistent with an overall government strategy of privatization.

It was not only pay rises that authorities were required to accommodate in their budgets but also improvements in service. For example, a report from the Maternity Services Advisory Committee (1985) highlighted services for very small, or ill, babies saying that 'Many regional centres are working under considerable strain with facilities which are (in the professionals' view) totally inadequate to meet the rising demand created by the prospects of the survival of more very small and ill babies'. This is an important comment on the impact of success in some areas then having cost implications in others.

The incidence of stillbirths and deaths in the very earliest period of life had gone down and credit for this was something the government quickly claimed. But such success does have implications for the next period of life. This is a realization that is important historically in that it further draws into focus the mistaken assumption in the establishment of the NHS that as it met fundamental health needs demand, and hence the need for expenditure, would reduce. The Minister, in accepting the critical report, said that all regional health authorities would be instructed to incorporate the Maternity Services Advisory Committee's advice in their strategic plans, but that money to implement the changes required would have to come from existing cash-limited budgets.

The improvements identified as being required would have to be made over a ten-year period, something that did not satisfy the pressure groups concerned with post-natal health services. They pointed to reports from doctors saying that about a third of all babies needing intensive care did not get it. King's College Hospital, London, was turning away 12–15 babies a month, University College five to ten a week and, according to a report to the House of Commons Social Services Committee, 30 per cent of babies needing intensive care in London could not be admitted to hospital (*Guardian*, 22 February 1985).

As well as the sale of assets and the strict enforcement of cash limits, whatever the identified need, the other device for trying to maintain the NHS without increasing government expenditure was to raise money directly by charges. On 1 April 1985 prescription charges went up to £2 per item. This new price represented a 1000 per cent increase since 1979. The increase in prescription charges from £1.60 would, it was estimated, raise another £19 million. This would help offset the loss of income from the part-privatization of opticians which would also come into effect on the same day. Dental charges were also going up by 25 per cent and a new way of calculating them would be introduced. NHS spectacles would now only be available to the poor, children, students and those who needed special glasses. Private patients' charges would go up by 14 per cent.

In an exchange in Parliament, when the increases were announced, the Secretary of State argued that considerably more was to be spent on the NHS in the coming year and that 'prescription charges had to make a contribution to that rise' (*Guardian*, 12 March 1985). Interestingly, it was being argued that increased income from higher charges represented part of the figure of increased expenditure, which the government would then take credit for!

The summer saw the regular reports of independent review bodies into nurses' and doctors' pay. The government partially accepted their recommendations but asserted that cash limits must be adhered to. Increases above these must be financed from the predetermined allocations. The government was seeking to abolish the concept of comparability in public pay and replace it with the watchword of affordability. To this they wished to add the market concept of pay being linked with recruitment potential (*Guardian*, 7 June 1985). This pay round saw the continuing juxtaposition of NHS pay increases (particularly for nurses) and financial problems for health authorities. The pay awards, which were indeed larger than the cash limits for inflation increases, could be offset to an extent by the privatization of ancillary services but many authorities had to contemplate funding them from cuts in services. One authority, Medway, announced that it was planning cuts of £1.1 million and these could include ward closures, ending the Family Planning Service, closing the only hospital on the Isle of Sheppey and cutting back on psychiatric and children's services (*Guardian*, 30 August 1985).

Nurses and midwives account for nearly half the NHS workforce with, at the end of 1983, the equivalent of 486,000 full-time staff including agency nurses. They cost £3487 million a year, almost 3 per cent of all public expenditure. Figures on the number of nurses employed suggested an increase of 16 per cent between 1976 and 1983 but this was in large part explained by new calculations which depended on a reduction in the number of working hours. A real staff increase in this period is better placed at around 6 per cent. This was at a time when there had been a 12 per cent increase in the number of hospital in-patients and a 7 per cent rise in out-patients. Again the figures are problematic in that they may reflect just shorter periods in hospital and more frequent readmissions rather than an increase in workload of the order they might at first glance suggest. But it was clear that there had been a more intensive use of acute beds and more hospital care for the very elderly, who are more dependent on nursing care.

It was with this scenario in mind that a National Audit Office report on nursing (Comptroller and Auditor General 1985) made recommendations about ways of achieving greater efficiency and so reducing expenditure on nursing. It commented that although many doctors complain of a lack of nursing presence this is to do with inefficiency in organization and particularly unequal distribution and not with an absolute shortage of numbers. For example, it pointed to a too generous overlap of nursing rosters. It suggested that there was a frequent failure to match the number of nurses on a ward with the number of patients and that the result was that there might be shortages in one area while another was over-staffed. It recommended closing wards at weekends, reorganizing shifts and redeploying staff and suggested that substantial savings could be made as a result. Action in the two latter areas alone, it argued, could save the 13 health authorities they studied between £2.3 million and £2.7 million.

It is certainly true that the nursing budget is very large and relatively minor changes in it can produce significant differences in expenditure. This is something well known to managers who may be slow at refilling nursing vacancies because keeping a number of unfilled posts over the year can give them a considerable flexibility in relocating the money they save. But it is also the case that a dimension other than the strict terms of an audit report is needed to understand the staffing needs of nursing. For example, a 'long' period of crossover on rosters may be necessary for the correct transmission of information about patients. It may allow a nurse who has experienced stress or upset during his or her shift to talk this through in such a way that it facilitates a better understanding of the patient's needs and allows the nurse to continue to do a difficult job without adding to the high numbers leaving the profession and so not 'repaying' the costs of their training.

As to closing wards at weekends, this presumably means that a person still has to be cared for and that it is most likely the caring will be done by the unpaid (and uncalculated) labour of their family, and usually of the women in their family. It is axiomatic that much of a so-called community care programme is, in reality, dependent upon the exploitation of the unpaid labour of women in the home (see, for example, Finch and Groves 1986; Land and Rose 1986). Discharge at weekends also ignores the adverse home circumstances many patients would be returned to, not least in terms of the quality of their housing. Information gained from audits and the policy advice linked to them needs to be evaluated in relation to the terms of reference of the audit.

If the organization of nursing was subject of scrutiny with a view to developing practice that would appear more efficient, in narrow cost terms, another subject of abiding concern – and of investigation – was the way health authorities rationed services through the use of waiting lists. A survey of 70 authorities found that in the 'worst' of them 72 per cent of patients were on waiting lists of over a year for general surgery while in the 'best' only 2 per cent were. Not only were there large differences between authorities but also between specialisms within the same authority; for example, Crewe had one of the worst waiting times in the country for general surgery but one of the shortest waiting times for orthopaedic. The report advised patients to exercise their right to have a GP refer them to an area where the waiting list was shorter (College of Health 1985), a response that might aid the more mobile but would do nothing for the problem of the relationship between identified need and available service throughout the country.

The year ended with continuing pressure to help health authorities with the implications of the nurses' pay award. It appeared that the combined approach of the Royal College of Nursing, the BMA, health administrators and health authorities to obtain some more funds to be able to meet the pay settlement without recourse to more attacks on services met with some success (*Guardian*, 8 November 1985).

As well as making concessions the government was also giving more attention to the presentation of policy. It planned an information pack to help health authority managers and chairmen counter criticisms of services. These criticisms were pronounced in London. The four largest Thames regions would lose 0.3 per cent in finance on the year's budget. The impact of the Resource Allocation Working Party (RAWP) formula was producing a number of acute problems. Examples included Bloomsbury District Health Authority's plans to close the Middlesex and University College Hospital to non-emergency patients for four weeks because the authority had exceeded its budget by £100 million; City and Hackney District Health Authority's plans to cut 10 per cent of its acute beds to help finance the year's pay rise for staff; and Hampstead District Health Authority's plans to cut spending by £1.4 million and to close wards (*Sunday Times*, 1 December 1985).

In 1986 the operation of the cash limits policy continued to have problems in terms of the lack of flexibility it built into the system. Three examples will illustrate. First, the drugs bill, despite the limited list, was increasing at approximately 7 per cent per year and less was being saved than had been hoped. The total annual NHS expenditure on drugs was approaching £2000 million and drug company profits remained high. Companies whose output was damaged by the limited list just made staff redundancies and maintained profitability for the company (*Guardian*, 11 February 1986). Second, the government, in its response to the fourth report from the Social Services Committee (DHSS 1986a), accepted a recommendation that more consultants be appointed, thereby adjusting a disparity between the number of non-consultant and consultant posts in the NHS. But this acceptance did not mean such a change would be funded. Third, and yet again, the problems associated with the nurses' pay claim and the flight of nurses from the profession did not seem solvable within the tight cash limits policy being applied. (As we have seen, 35 per cent of nurses give up before completing training and a further 33 per cent later resign from the profession (House of Commons Committee of Public Accounts 1986a).) The DHSS estimated that during 1986 the number of nurses employed in the NHS would fall by 2000 and this they attributed to recruitment problems.

As well as being critical of the level of pay and of the cuts in services which had been linked with financing the nurses' previous pay increase nursing leaders pointed out the changing nature of NHS activity. It had changed, they argued, from a service based on cure to one where the emphasis was on care. This was a direct result of changes in the characteristics of likely recipients of the service, both in terms of age and of the chronic presenting problems that are associated with this demographic change (Sheila Quinn, President of the Royal College of Nursing, quoted in the *Guardian*, 29 April 1986).

The year 1986 also saw the by now familiar debates about the real nature of NHS expenditure. There might now be a shared recognition that expenditure must increase by more than inflation in order even to keep pace with demographic and technological factors, but the extent of the required increase and where this extra money should come from – either increased funding or efficiency savings – remained at the centre of debate.

Cash limits meant that costs that rose more than the limits allowed would have to be met from the ongoing allocation. But the situation was made more complex by the way increased costs were calculated. For example the pay increases announced in May did exceed the cash limits although the extent to which they did was moderated by the device of deferring a part of the agreed increase until 1 July. Nurses' pay was to rise by an average of 7.8 per cent but because that award was defered until 1 July (as opposed to the start of the financial year in April) the real value of the year's increase was 5.9 per cent. Doctors and dentists were to get an average of 7.6 per cent but, because of the deferment, effectively got 5.7 per cent. General and unit managers' pay was to go up by between 3.5 per cent and 7.5 per cent. They were to be subject to a greater emphasis on performance-related pay. All security of tenure in general management was abolished and replaced with rolling short-term contracts. District general managers were to receive between £28,800 and £31,600 and unit managers between £15,600 and £26,400. Regional general managers' pay was fixed at £33,200 (*Guardian*, 23 May 1986).

The other abiding problem which returned to the centre of attention in June 1986 was cuts in central London hospitals. They reported particularly severe problems associated with the RAWP redistributions. The leaders of 12 teaching hospitals came together jointly to publicize their plight. Twenty inner London hospitals and 2,500 beds had been lost. Waiting lists were 675,000 strong, with 150,000 of these people waiting for over a year. Some hospitals were in severe states of disrepair; St Thomas's estimated that its maintenance backlog would cost £1.7 million to remedy. There was a severe lack of modern equipment and the impact of this was that some people's lives would be needlessly shortened. Further, morale was very low, affected by the conditions of work including pay (*Guardian*, 10 June 1986).

The picture these hospitals were presenting was a very serious one and certainly was considered in the DHSS to have potential electoral consequences. The Secretary of State sought leave from the Treasury to increase the money spent on health in the forthcoming spending round and in particular to allocate funds to enable waiting lists to be cut (*Guardian*, 16 June 1986).

These events are in themselves good indicators of the politics of health and of the distribution of power and influence. The concerted efforts of pressure groups and concerned parties, both behind the scenes and in public, raised the issue to prominence. Coincident with the Press coverage, a TV programme, *World in Action* (Granada Television, 9 June 1986), named patients whose deaths could, it claimed, be directly attributed to health cuts. These claims were taken up by the Labour Party, which clearly saw them as offering a series of specific and well-supported criticisms of the government's position that changes in health finances were being implemented without damage to patient services. Also gaining widespread recognition was a perception that the government's record on the NHS would be of major importance in any forthcoming general election and that that election was likely to occur within the time-span of the next spending round. Together these factors gave the Secretary of State a strong hand in his negotiations. We can assume, as I have argued in an earlier chapter, that additionally he saw arguing for increased expenditure on health services as consistent with his interests at this time.

Waiting lists were clearly being targeted by the government for action. Each regional health authority was asked by the DHSS to investigate them. The review, they were told, did not mean that extra funds would be forthcoming although their results 'would be closely scrutinised'. Opportunities for even more efficiency savings should be investigated. The record on efficiency savings was that in 1984–5 £105 million, in 1985–6 £153 million, and an anticipated £150 million in 1986–7, had been achieved (House of Commons Committee of Public Accounts 1986b). The lessons of good practice needed to be passed on – 20 of the 190 health districts accounted for a quarter of all hospital waiting list numbers (*Guardian*, 22 July 1986).

As well as the encouragement to change practice the other tactic used, again a familiar one, was to present some alternative figures. In August the DHSS *Statistical Bulletin* (2/1986) reported that a record number of patients had been treated in 1985, despite a fall in the number of beds. The number of in-patients treated was 6.35 million, 176,000 more than in 1984, and nearly a million more than in 1978. Out-patient cases rose by 398,000 to 37.4 million and day cases were up to 60,000 to 963,000. Over a period of ten years the number of patients treated per bed had risen by almost a half. The average length of stay in hospital had dropped to 7.6 days (down by 0.2 days). Geriatric departments had treated more patients, hospital day attendances for mental illness had gone up by 111,000 to 3.4 million and the average number of occupied beds had fallen by 2000, reflecting the trend away from in-patient care.

As with all such sets of figures, their publication prompted alternative analyses of their meaning. One critic, Lord David Ennals (a former Labour minister), pointed to the figures on increases in in-patient treatment as reflecting not more people being treated but more admissions and readmissions, the same people being counted more than once.

If more and more was being spent then it was not the 24 per cent more that the government claimed but rather the figure presented by the all-party House of Commons Select Committee, which concluded that between 1980–1 and 1985–6 real spending on hospital and community services, in constant price terms, had increased by 2.2 cent, or 0.4 per cent per year. When that is put alongside the general agreement that spending needs to increase by 2 per cent per year to keep pace one can clearly see what is well known to the providers of the service – that there is an actual cut in budgets and consequent service reduction. The Select Committee concluded that 'the most telling way of representing the shortfall is to say that between 1980/1 and 1985/6 the cumulative under-funding of the hospital and community health services current account was £1325 billion at 1985/6 prices' (letter to the *Guardian*, 20 August 1986).

As long as there are such fundamental disputes about the reality of spending figures the actual picture is difficult to identify. The politics of presentation is of considerable importance not just because it helps hide what each side wishes to hide but because whoever wins this particular struggle takes the initiative, defines the parameters of debate and makes the other side appear destructive and petty.

A number of commentators on party politics in the United Kingdom have identified the need for the Left to break out of a political agenda defined by the Right. They observe the dynamism in terms of generating ideas about social change as coming from the Right. This leaves the Left defending ground of which it might well have been critical in other circumstances. In relation to policy on health, housing and education, Hilary Wainwright (1987, pp. 44–5) argues for a politics of 'relationism' to counter both the individualism of the Right (fast being embraced by Neil Kinnock and the Labour Party, she suggests) and the collectivism of the previous Left position. The concentration ought to be on the democracy of social provision and its responsiveness to varying needs. Eric Hobsbawm (1987) has also argued for some time for the need to reappraise the politics of the Left in such a way that the initiative can be once again seized: 'The reason why we have not made headway against Thatcherism is that Thatcherism is still the only programme on offer with the object of changing the British economy.' He is arguing for a politics in which the argument for alternative forms of both economic and social organization is vigorously pursued and in which old forms are not simply defended but scrutinized, criticized and where necessary discarded (Hosbawm 1987, p. 19).

We have to add to the argument about figures the complex debate on the impact of the efficiency saving programme. It ought, theoretically, to be possible if such a programme is successful both to improve services and not to increase expenditure. The Secretary of State in September, when the next round of negotiations about pay and funding began, argued that health authorities in England had achieved £150 million savings from their cost improvements in the previous year. This was the equivalent of a 1.5 per cent increase in their resources. A similar saving was being planned in the current year. Thus with this, and with the small increase in absolute funding, the 'extra funding' of over 2 per cent to enable the NHS to stay the same was exceeded and the NHS consequently was in real terms, in the sense of usable funding and service to patients, improving. There were three issues in dispute here. The first was one of substantive fact. Had these efficiency savings been made or were they merely reductions in service called something else? Second, and allied with this, had 'efficiency savings' been audited in such a way that any deleterious impact on patient services was calculated? Third, even if they had been achieved, had the scope for more savings now disappeared?

A report prepared at York University's Centre for Health Economics, as well as contributing to the considerable speculation about the true nature of spending increases, pointed to the absence of evidence about the costs and effects of alternative ways of providing community care for any of the targeted groups. The emphasis on making decisions designed to save money is therefore being made without adequate information on real cost or on efficacy and outcome (*Guardian*, 2 September 1986).

These observations link with Professor Williams of York seeking to develop means of comparing costs and outcomes of treatments. He told the British Association annual meeting in September 1986 that kidney dialysis was one of the most expensive forms of medical treatment and hip replacement one of the cheapest in terms of improved quality of life and that we 'should not shrink from following where the logic of that approach leads us – that hospital dialysis should be restrained and total hip replacement expanded' (reported in the *Guardian*, 4 September 1986). The logic of that approach could lead some of us to a different conclusion, we may seek to improve the total allocation of funds so that both treatments can be carried out, or we may want to question why dialysis is so expensive and look at the profits of drug companies and medical equipment manufacturers. Other concerns about the long-term impact of efficiency savings and the sale of assets were also voiced at the British Association, where such measures were described as akin to 'selling the furniture to pay the rent'.

The government's decision to target waiting lists for concentrated attention appeared to have some localized impact. The NHS Management Centre directed its attention to the West Midlands and Wales and managed to reduce the number on waiting lists considerably. They first checked if everyone on the list still wanted the service. Some had died and some had opted for private treatment. Then they targeted resources in such a way as to make a maximum impact on the waiting list. With finite resources this meant that a decision was made that the reduction of the lists was paramount, a decision certainly emanating from the consideration of the political damage of long lists. Labour's health spokesman, Frank Dobson, said that he had evidence that health authorities had been switching resources to quick and simple operations to hold down their waiting lists at the expense of more complex, time-consuming, cases.

If improvements had been made in some areas the national picture was that over the year little impact had been made on the total number of people on waiting lists. There were still major anomalies; for example, half the ear, nose and throat beds in the country were empty while a quarter of ear, nose and throat patients had to wait over a year for admission. One further note on waiting times: the College of Health complained that the government had collected figures from health authorities in March but had not passed them on to the public until September (*Guardian*, 9 October 1986)!

Once again the basis of the figures and the implications attributed to them are not straightforward. There is a difference between waiting times and waiting lists; the latter had increased from 661,249 to 673,107 in the year up to September, whereas the former had fallen marginally. In March 1986 24 per cent of non-urgent cases had been waiting more than a year compared with 24.2 per cent in September 1985. Consequently government spokesmen concentrated on times and the Opposition and other critics on lists (*Guardian*, 25 November 1986). Some health authorities were experiencing significant increases in the number on waiting lists for urgent treatment. These included North-West Thames Region, up by 21.2 per cent; North-East Thames up by 20.4 per cent; and, outside London, North-Western Region, 16.3 per cent; and Merseyside 11.6 per cent (London Health Emergency 1986).

1987 did not bring essentially new arguments, though as it was to be an election year the emphasis did change. As well as the findings of the London Health Emergency study the capital was under close scrutiny from a study commissioned by the King's Fund. London had already lost three-quarters of the acute beds it was destined to lose by 1993 but health authorities had only achieved a third of their savings targets. At the heart of the overall planning cycle for 1983–93 was the reduction of the numbers of beds in London and the redistribution of the released money to the NHS outside London. But the problem was that the demand for beds in the capital continued to increase and the reduction in beds was anyway not going to allow authorities to meet the savings targets. The London region's long-term plans included an assumption of a 15 per cent cut in inner London hospital admissions over the planning period. In fact there was a 2.5 per cent increase in in-patients and a 6 per cent increase in out-patients during 1983–5 (bear in mind the problems of defining what a patient actually is, as described above). The dilemma for health authorities was summed up by the Chairman of the City and Hackney District Health Authority, who pointed out that it was not cost effective to reduce activity by 20 per cent to make savings of 5 per cent (King's Fund Institute 1987). The Minister of Health, Tony Newton, stated his belief that the report gave an incomplete picture and, in particular, did not acknowledge a 'bridging fund' of £30 million over two years would largely benefit the inner London districts (*Guardian*, 20 January 1987).

One solution to the problem of linking the allocation of resources to an immediate improvement in service is to target specifically and direct centrally. The decision to direct extra funds at shortening waiting lists was a good example of such a process. Not only was the DHSS giving extra money for a priority it, rather than the health authorities, had specified but it was specifically directing the first £25 million of what would be an eventual £50 million package to provide certain kinds of operation. For example Bloomsbury health district in London, with the longest waiting list in the country, would get £200,000 for 170 joint replacement operations: Trent region's £2.4 million would mean treatment for 1200 children in ear, nose and throat clinics. It was planned that 100,000 people from the waiting lists could be treated as a result of this initiative (*Guardian*, 18 February 1987).

The plan reputedly came from Sir Roy Griffiths and included, in true Griffiths style, a requirement that authorities report back and that progress be closely scrutinized. It was a very centralized system and somewhat at odds with the principle of managerial independence at local level. But, as Frank Dobson observed, it had to be seen in the context of an anticipated general election.

Closely linked with a prioritization of reducing waiting lists and of being more cost effective and efficient was a concern with how long patients stay in hospital. The length of time spent in hospital had gone down; in one hospital, for example, the length of in-patient treatment following a Caesarean section had been reduced from 14 to eight days and for a hysterectomy from 21 to eight days. Faster throughput may aid the figures on treatment and on waiting lists but its critics claim it gives primacy to financial rather than medical efficiency (*Observer*, 1 February 1987). It also once again includes the possibility of hidden non–audited costs either in the greater possibility of readmission or in a diversion of care into other sectors, particularly the utilization of the unpaid domestic labour of women carers.

Most concern was centred on cuts in the NHS, but the actual state of the health of the population had been the subject of reports commissioned by the Health Education Council (HEC) before its demise. We have already looked at the update of the Black Report on inequalities in health. The second report on child health jointly commissioned by the HEC and the National Children's Bureau was completed in March 1987 although the date of publication was to be July 1987 (National Children's Bureau 1987).

This report updated the Court Report (DHSS 1976b) on child health services and was prepared by Professor Philip Graham, Dean of the Institute of Child Health. The Court Report had called for an improvement of services to ensure that the right care was available for children of all ages. This was far from being achieved. There was a considerable disparity between the amount of resources districts devoted to child health, some spending five times more than others. The quality of the school health service had declined, as had school meals. The NHS reorganization of 1982 had abolished area medical and nursing officers, the people responsible for the co-ordination of children's health, and there were still no community paediatricians to take over (*Guardian*, 27 March 1987).

The final report of the HEC was to be on preventive health where it was predicted a decline in services would be identified. The three HEC reports were important in that each served to remind that a health service is not hermetically sealed and that events in the broader society contribute centrally to the state of the nation's health.

But in the more specific area of the treatment of illness the kinds of choice being made by the NHS remained often hidden and certainly not the subject of public debate. Kidney specialists in the Renal Association, and in conjunction with the British Diabetic Association, had been researching the practice of discriminating, in making decisions about the possibilities of kidney dialysis or organ transplant, against the over-45s and against those with complications like diabetes. One consultant, Dr Gwyn Williams, believed that the implication of this was that every year up to 500 diabetics who were suffering from kidney failure, but who could be saved, were turned away to die. There are 1,265,000 diabetics in the United Kingdom, 2 per cent of the population, and approximately 630,000 of them already have, or will develop, kidney problems of varying seriousness. The likelihood of being offered treatment appeared to depend on GP referral and then on hospitals having the facilities to offer help. Because of a shortage of facilities for treatment, not because such treatment is more difficult or less likely to be successful if you suffer from these complaints, it will be an accident of geography and of age that will determine if you live or die (*Guardian*, 29 April 1987).

It would not be realistic to argue that such decisions were new ones, although the advances in medical technology do make it more likely that people could live, given certain treatments. Nor is it the case that one can deny the apparently infinite demands that could be made on a health service and the problem of allocating finite resources. But who makes the decision, on what grounds and with what legitimacy? The sorts of decision might include one that says if you are older than 45 and have kidney problems then you are too old to be worth offering help. Even if we adopt Professor Williams's QALYs, or a DHSS variation of them, surely we have to argue about the overall level of funding appropriate to a health service and not just the manipulation of limited funds between competing interests within it. It is not something that should be subject either to medical discretion or to the calculator logic of instrumental reason.

As well as the treatment offered to its patients we must consider the way the NHS utilizes its staff. We have seen how, either explicitly or implicitly, the needs of staff have been set into opposition against those of patients and prospective patients through arguments on the impact pay claims have on cash-limited authorities. Two examples of the impact of government policy on staff will illustrate further problems. They are from very different settings.

One hundred and fifty professors of medicine offered their opinions on the state of medical research to the House of Lords Science and Technology Committee. The picture they presented was one of 'rock bottom morale and very poor recruitment'. The number of university-funded posts had been cut by 15 per cent since 1981 and the number of clinical medical academic staff had fallen from 2165 in 1979 to 1728 in 1984. A statement in reply was made in the House of Lords by the government's Junior Health Minister, Baroness Trumpington. She said that the number of full-time staff in the universities had been increased in this period. A reading of the staffing figures can produce both, conflicting, results. Extra people were in the main on short-term contracts, mostly funded by the drug industry or by charities. They were working on very specifically delineated projects and not the sort of work that would be considered fundamental, either clinically or biologically. Such projects are usually directed towards the solution of a problem in the here and now rather than the pursuit of 'purer' research where the practical implications are not apparent at the time the research is being done.

Each sort of research will have its uses. But in a system that is dependent on commercial sponsorship the likelihood is that targeted research to identify particular marketable products will take precedence and when such a possibility does not exist research will not be funded. Charities are often in a similar position in that they have to attract funds by offering tangible results arising from their spending. Three examples of likely problems will illustrate. First, if a product does not look as if it will reap a big financial reward it is not pursued. Such is the case with the attempts to develop a new anti malarial drug – soon to be crucial for the health of large numbers in Africa and Asia. But such a drug, for which demand comes from poor countries, does not promise a high return on investment and so that investment has not materialized and the drug is not being developed (Prof. Wallace Peters, *World at One*, BBC Radio 4, 8 June 1987). Second, in research into AIDS the emphasis will be on producing a drug that can be quickly marketable. Because of that the pursuit of alleviating symptoms will take precedence over the more speculative long-term development of knowledge about the body's immune system. But it is the latter which would enable the syndrome to be understood, eradicated and which would leave us better equipped to respond to any similar scenario in the future (Small 1988). Third, if research initiatives are left to industry non-drug-related research such as preventive medicine and epidemiology will not be funded. Some specialisms might not receive the attention they require because they are not seen as being susceptible to dramatic interventions and the creation of a lucrative market for any developed product. Research in general medicine will also be distorted in that it will be shifted away from methods of diagnosis and treatment that are not based on drugs (*Guardian*, 14 May 1987).

Paradoxically, as well as the impacts on the long-term future of research and scientific development in Britain, the other result of leaving much initiative in funding research to drug companies is that the NHS is likely to be offered the results of these endeavours in the form of a new series of high-priced drugs which will swell its huge drugs bill. The policy of short-term savings may therefore have an impact not just on the effectiveness of the service but also on its longer-term cost.

The second example of the impact of the government's policy on the staff of the NHS involves looking at the situation in district general hospitals (and the hospital service more generally). A survey in the *Observer* (3 May 1987) identified the three most common complaints from hospital staff as being a shortage of nurses particularly in specialized fields like theatre nursing, intensive care and geriatrics; a shortage of back-up staff like secretaries, laboratory staff and therapists of all sorts; and a shortage of junior doctors, most notably in orthopaedics, paediatrics and accident and emergency departments. In the first two categories low pay and overwork were blamed for a lack of recruits. The situation of junior doctors was linked with three factors. General practice had become more popular than hospital work. The Department of Health strictly limited the number of junior doctors to try and ensure that there were not too many juniors looking for senior jobs as consultants (the relationship between numbers of consultants and of juniors had been recently altered to increase the proportion of consultants). New immigration rules had resulted in a dramatic drop in the number of overseas doctors seeking posts in British hospitals.

Some consequences of these problems are illustrative of the more fundamental dilemmas of staffing in the contemporary NHS. One of the areas of greatest progress medically is in neo-natal care, but the demands such units impose on their staff are considerable. They are the hardest units to staff in the hospital and there appears a constant shortage of nurses (*Observer Magazine*, 18 October 1987). The improvements technically mean that many babies who would have died in the recent past do not now die, but not all survive, of course. The neo-natal unit has to cope with the stresses of nursing the very sick and weak and dealing with hugely insecure and anxious families. It has to help parents establish relationships with babies not just in a very public environment but in one so foreign to their expectations. It also has to deal with the inevitable deaths and with the discovery that some children will live but will be physically and/or brain-damaged. (The long-term emotional impact on parent and child of early care in such a unit is speculated about but not widely theorized or researched.) The planning and resource dilemma, therefore, is that one has to understand neo-natal care as being far more than an environment for technological flair. It has to be properly resourced and supported as a caring environment.

Two more specific examples of the problems of neo-natal care and paediatrics came to public attention in 1987. In May the Brompton Hospital, London, had eight paediatric intensive care cots occupied. Though the recommended nursing cover for these was one nurse per cot, there were only four nurses available. There were not enough nurses specialized in paediatrics and intensive care to allow the hospital to operate on other babies in urgent need and two such referrals had to be transferred to the nearby private Cromwell Hospital where they were given emergency operations, paid for by the NHS (*Guardian*, 29 May 1987). Earlier in the year a 17-bed unit at Stoke Mandeville Hospital, which provided operations within the first 48 hours of life for babies born with cleft lips and palates, was closed down for two months to save money. The benefit of operating at such an early stage is that babies heal more quickly and are less likely to suffer defects later in life. This also saves the NHS money in the longer term, as well as saving families considerable distress and uncertainty. But the costing policy is such that long-term benefits (or human benefits) cannot be offset against the problems for this particular unit as it exceeds its cash limit for the year (*Guardian*, 29 January 1987).

There are other absurdities created by staff shortages and the imposition of cash and personnel limits. As we have noted above, the two sorts of control may not coincide in their impact on the actual service. Dewsbury district, in Yorkshire, reported spending £1000 a week on hiring locums to fill the post of paediatric registrar because it was not allowed to fill the post on a permanent basis (*Observer*, 3 May 1987).

Although the general election intervened the general trend of concern about the impact of cash limits on services continued. Waiting lists remained high despite the Secretary of State's extra targeted funding, and regional variations were considerable. A College of Health (1987) report provided the most up-to-date figures. At the end of September 1986, 724,350 people were on NHS waiting lists, a 3 per cent increase on 1985 figures. Some people waited up to four years for 'non-urgent' operations (sometimes to get an out-patient appointment just to get on an operating list can take a considerable time – it was not unknown for hapless patients to turn up on the right date except that they were a year early!). In 29,145 urgent cases (including those where there was a possibility of a diagnosis of cancer), the patient had been waiting more than a month.

One commentator, himself a former NHS administrator (Yates, 1987), suggested that the practice of consultants needed to be closely examined and evaluated. Perhaps, he argued, NHS administrators and consultants should be penalized for long waiting lists and patients compensated. Consultants vary considerably in the number of operations they carry out and this disparity should be the subject of scrutiny. It was a suggestion not inconsistent with the spirit of the Griffiths reforms. He suggested this be linked with a study of the place of private practice. Two new additions to the mythology of the NHS are that you can get an operation privately tomorrow for which you would have to wait years on the NHS, and that consultants are not unhappy about long waiting lists because it is these that are the recruiting ground for private practice. Yates wonders if for consultants 'the failure to cope with an NHS workload can be financially advantageous'.

Spending on private health care has grown four times faster than spending on the NHS, according to an Office of Health Economics research report (OHE 1987). In 1981 it had exceeded £1 billion. Three hundred NHS hospitals had closed and the total number of available beds had fallen by 15 per cent. The report calculated that this had meant a total underfunding of the NHS by £900 million since 1980. This report was interesting, not so much for the figures it presented – they were well known – but because of its source. The OHE is the drug industry's research body and the industry is among the Conservative Party's biggest financial supporters. The report's conclusions were not in accord with the position the government was advancing about the state of the NHS in the 1980s. This does suggest that the industry was concerned that a decline in the NHS might adversely effect profits from the sale of existing drugs and the development of new ones.

The report argued that the NHS had failed to keep pace with the cost of medical advances, pay rises and the rising demand from the increasing number of elderly people. Even though £22.4 billion was spent on health care in 1986 (just under £400 per person), representing 6.1 per cent of UK Gross National Product, these figures still left the United Kingdom behind many other industrialized countries. Taking into account wage and price inflation the report suggested that resources had risen in volume terms by 26 per cent since 1973. That increase was not evenly distributed among the regions; for example, North-West Thames and South-West Thames had lost 6 per cent and 2 per cent, respectively, during the decade. The proportion of NHS spending that went on hospitals had decreased from 62 per cent in 1975 to 58 per cent in 1986. The report concluded from these figures that

> Hospital spending has risen by one per cent a year in volume terms since 1980, one half less than the target growth needed to keep pace with rising demand from the increasing number of elderly people and medical advances, as well as to meet the Government's policy objectives.

Hence the cumulative total underfunding figure of £900 million between 1980 and 1986.

The GP service, which was only nominally cash-limited, increased its share of the NHS budget in the same period. There were a record 32,355 GPs in the NHS in 1985 and the number of consultations was estimated to have risen by 9 per cent in the decade to 249 million in 1986 (the equivalent of 4.4 consultations per year per person). The GP drugs bill more than doubled from £919 million in 1979 to just under £2 billion in 1986. Drugs accounted for about 10 per cent of NHS spending although that still represented a smaller expenditure per head than in many Western European and Scandinavian countries. Rises in the drugs bill were explained by the increased demands of the elderly (remember who is doing this research) with the average elderly person being given 15 prescription items in 1986.

Figures from the hospital sector are more problematic (as we have discovered). Hospital manpower rose by 13 per cent to nearly a million over the decade to 1986. Doctors, midwives and nurses accounted for the majority of this increase. But this magnitude of increase was an increase on paper and not in terms of personnel because it was based on a different way of calculating the figures. The number of in-patients also increased by 27 per cent during the decade to a record 7.9 million in 1985, though, as we have seen, this reflects different dominant practices in admission and discharge policy.

As well as this report on the state of the NHS and its finances a number more were in preparation. The King's Fund was looking into private sector finance and collaboration with the NHS. The Institute of Health Service Management was also seeking to review organization and finance so that it could avoid seeing the NHS 'bleed to death by a thousand cuts' as its President put it. The Public Expenditure Policy Unit (a think tank headed by a former deputy secretary of finance at the DHSS) was looking at, among other things, how much public resistance there would be to user charges, for example for specialist services, to see a GP or be admitted to hospital. One way of combining a solution to under-funding on the one hand and considerable public support for more resources to be spent on the NHS, they suggested, might be to get people who used the services to pay (*Guardian*, 14 September 1987).

One group which had already gone public with some suggestions was the Institute of Economic Affairs (IEA 1987). The IEA presented for discussion the possibility of making patients pay for the drugs they had prescribed and allowing the drug companies to charge whatever the market could take (those on supplementary benefit would be exempt). It argued that the resulting increase in drug company profits would result in more jobs, more exports, greater innovation and greater efficiency. Further it would improve surgery relationships because instead of the doctor handing down instructions from on high both doctor and patient together would have to consider options and the cost of treatment.

6 Privatization

Private enterprise has always been an important component of the NHS. A considerable proportion of the funds given to the NHS is then paid out to the private sector via drug and equipment bills. Also, from its inception, private practice has existed alongside the NHS. This was something that had been fought for by the doctors and was of both economic and symbolic importance (which of these was dominant has varied over time). But in recent years the extent of privatization and its importance in the present and in visions of the future for the NHS have increased considerably.

I will begin my review of developments with a *Which?* report on private medical insurance from June 1984 (*Which?* 1984). Much of the literature from private health firms draws prospective customers' attention to the shortcomings of the NHS. These they identify as endless waiting lists, no privacy and lack of individual attention. They contrast this with private medical care, which is presented as being speedy, efficient and carried out in cheerful, modern and private surroundings. The private sector concentrated on the treatment of non-urgent surgical conditions for which there were long waiting lists, such as hernias and varicose veins. In 1984 there were 8000 beds in private hospitals and in addition there were 3000 pay beds in NHS hospitals. This represented a total that was still under 5 per cent of surgical beds available under the NHS. But they had targeted areas with long waiting lists. For example the average waiting time in NHS hospitals for a varicose vein operation was between 20 and 55 weeks depending on which part of the country the patient lived in. For hernias it was between 15 and 25 weeks.

The stereotyped image of the NHS presented in the publicity material of private companies may be true in part but it is not the whole picture. Not all NHS patients are treated in huge impersonal wards, for example. Private hospitals may not have the kinds of specialized equipment, or the back-up personnel, to cope with emergencies. Costs of treatment can be considerable but then premiums for medical insurance are also high. If you paid BUPA's lowest scale for people living outside London and contributed to the scheme from age 18 to age 65, at present rates, you would have paid £9779; on the top rate and in London the amount paid would be £18,529. Given, as in all insurance schemes, that most people do not make major claims perhaps it would be more sound financial sense to put the premiums in a building society, accumulate interest, and hope you never have to draw on them.

It is often difficult to know what the total cost of an operation will be in advance. Complications can arise and consultants can charge the fees they think the patient will pay. Insurance companies, as warrants the free market, vary considerably in the premiums they charge and in the service they offer. But BUPA dominates with 70 per cent of the market. Their cover is not all-embracing, indeed there are a considerable number of things not included. They certainly do not appear to encourage older people to join; older people make more demands on health resources, after all. Premiums for those in the scheme who reach 65 are high; and there is no 'family reduction'. You can not join the ordinary scheme if you are 65 or over.

Pay beds, private hospitals and health insurance are only one part of the involvement of the private sector in the provision of health care. There is also the role of private industry in providing drugs and equipment, the increasing encouragement to seek outside contractors to provide services, for example laundry and cleaning in place of in-house labour, and the increase in charges at the point of use, most notably via prescriptions but also in dental and optician charges.

Most of the Press attention regarding these subjects seemed to centre on the mistakes and apparent absurdities of the system. For example, the private hospital that treated the Prime Minister's eye in 1983 apparently had to borrow NHS equipment to enable it to carry out the operation. There was no waiting list for eye operations in the Prime Minister's district but she preferred to have private treatment (*Guardian*, 7 March 1984).

Another item to excite Press interest was attempts to charge overseas visitors for NHS services, an innovation the government believed would raise £6 million in a year but which proved administratively impossible. One East Anglian hospital observed that they had issued five bills, only one of which, for £4.50, had been paid, and that they had spent £280 on stationery and £450 on staff time. NALGO estimated that the total collected nationally had been £374,459, but the cost of doing this was not known (*Guardian*, 27 February 1984).

The situation was becoming a serious one for NHS ancillary staff as pressure developed to move towards privatizing cleaning and laundry services. Such moves were presented as being part of a cost control exercise, the pursuit of greater cost effectiveness. But they also seemed to be encouraged by politicians as a policy initiative above and beyond the cost imperative. It did appear that the wish was not just to lower costs but also to lower the number of workers directly employed by the NHS. There were, therefore, two agendas that would not always coincide and privatization certainly provides rich grounds for speculation about the relative importance of the political, ideological and economic. A major debate about laundry services in Cornwall illustrated all these issues.

The essence of the Cornwall dispute was that the Minister directed the health authority to hire a private firm despite the existence of a lower tender from the existing workforce. The latter had put in an offer based on an acceptance by the workers of a pay cut and changes in some working practices. Not only did the government direct the acceptance of an offer that was not the lowest, and in so doing appear to contradict its own advice, but it was also acting against the wishes of both the Cornwall District Health Authority and the South Western Regional Health Authority, both Conservative-controlled and headed by chairmen appointed by the Secretary of State. The health authorities' opposition was on grounds of price and quality of service and was based on what was considered an unsatisfactory experience of the firm in question providing laundry service for one hospital in the region. The in-house tender would have saved £47,320 per year and avoided the loss of 40 jobs, and with them redundancy payments of £24,000.

Despite the authorities urging the Minister to let the in-house tender be considered in accordance with what they understood to be his own instructions, the Minister would not give way. Eventually the regional administrator spelled out the possible consequences of the authorities continuing to oppose the Minister. He would be able to 'persuade and lean' on authorities and if that were not successful he could take powers to ensure his instructions were followed. These could include removing the chairman and members of the authority. The contract was given to the private firm (*Guardian*, 23 March 1984).

If the Cornwall experience reminds us of ministerial power and the primacy of political considerations it is also important in giving an insight into the relative powerlessness of NHS workers in opposing privatization without worsening their own conditions of service. In September 1983 the government abolished Fair Wages Regulations. These had been accepted as forming part of the standing orders of health authorities and had meant that outside contractors had to offer pay and conditions of Whitley Council standard. This was no longer the case and hence both private and in-house contractors could offer to worsen conditions of service to help either win contracts or preserve jobs. This worsening starts from a low point anyway in terms of pay. Private firms might maintain the official NHS hourly rate (£1.64 in 1984 for domestic cleaners) but cut working hours, scrap weekend pay and reduce both personnel and time allocated for particular jobs. In Barking Hospital 90 National Union of Public

Employees (NUPE) cleaners were involved in a long strike precipitated by the private contracting cleaning firm offering new contracts which essentially meant a 40 per cent cut in hours and hence in earnings. In Leeds the number of full-time jobs attached to a new hospital wing was cut from 87 to 27 with the remainder of the work to be done by part-time labour.

There has been resistance to the government's privatization policy both from workers and from authorities. Some of the latter have refused, or delayed, compliance with the DHSS Circular ((83)18) instructing them to test all their services through competitive tender and report back via regions to the DHSS. Others have voted to reinstate Fair Wages clauses abolished by the government. Trade unions have publicly been opposed to privatization but appear aware of a mood among their members, which they attribute to the failure of the nine-month pay strike in 1982, making them reluctant to take major industrial action. In the main their tactic has been to offer support to workers in dispute (although no leadership, some members complain) and to pursue an educational policy. This has concentrated on running stewards' courses and encouraging trade union representatives to be involved in all stages in moves towards privatization and in the workplace thereafter (Cohen and Anderson 1984; see also Cohen 1984a).

It may be that the government's justification for privatization is to provide as good a service or better at a lower cost to the Exchequer, although the Cornish experience does not support this. But another result is that the workforce is more flexible in the sense that the NHS has commitments to less workers. Hence the possibility of making further cuts via another reduction in the workforce is made easier. At the same time the power of trade unions is diminished and workers' rights and standards of employment eroded.

Health Circular (83)18 was a step towards the government's aim of increasing the proportion of the NHS provided by private enterprise to something approaching 25 per cent. A considerable number of firms would then be involved. One likely significant contributor was the Pritchard Services Group. This was the largest company operating in the NHS in 1984. It is a multinational company with an annual turnover of £300 million. It had lobbied both the Conservative Medical Society Symposium and the 1982 Conservative Party Conference, mounting an elaborate public relations exercise aimed at party activists. Pritchard's world-wide health interests did not just include cleaning. In the United States it runs Kimberley Nurses which provides temporary nurses to hospitals and nursing homes. In the United Kingdom it is very closely linked with BUPA, which is a major Pritchard shareholder. Clearly private enterprises see a considerable scope in many NHS activities for their involvement and for profit-making (Beckett 1984).

But privatization is not just the simple encroachment of private firms. In some instances non-profit-making charities are taking over NHS activities. The Kidney Research Unit Foundation (KRUF) has taken over the provision of dialysis in Wales. It promised to end the undoubtedly preventable loss of life associated with dialysis in the United Kingdom, which was twenty-first in the European league table of dialysis treatment per million of the population; it was calculated that there were 2000 premature and preventable deaths in the UK annually. In parts of the UK dialysis machines are in such short supply that doctors have to decide who lives and who dies. The practice has developed of giving priority to wage earners who have families to support. Critics of the British practice point to other countries where such decisions – one German doctor called them 'death committee decisions' – do not have to be made and dialysis can be given to those who need it. KRUF intended to run new dialysis centres which would be open six days a week with opening hours that allowed people with jobs to attend. The centres would have small specialized teams of nurses and, it was anticipated, operate at about half the annual costs of dialysis in hospitals (Iverson 1984).

There was an interesting twist to discussions about privatization in June 1984 when it was revealed that the investment fund managers for Sheffield District Health Authority had invested £95,000 in British American Tobacco and in Distillers. They argued that they had a responsibility to act in the best interests of the fund's eventual beneficiaries and that their concern was not with health as such. They cited the National Coal Board pension fund including in its portfolio gas and oil interests (*Guardian*, 2 June 1984).

The government's moves towards privatization seemed to be faltering and certainly were winning it few friends. It had critics from the Right; the Tory Reform Group proclaimed that the moves to privatize domestic services had been a failure and should be taken out of the hands of the health authorities and put under the control of a central unit. The government had been increasingly interventionist in the pursuit of this policy both in terms of issuing instructions to put out cleaning, catering and laundry to private tender and requiring progress reports by a fixed date. This was strengthened by a Circular (HC(83)18) setting down a detailed timetable. The Secretary of State had added pressure by making it known that he was interested in, and would encourage, experiment with private contractors in other fields such as estate management, transport and vehicle maintenance. He had also been prepared to intervene directly even against the wishes of health authorities, as we have seen in Cornwall. Yorkshire region and within that Calderdale district had also received unwanted instructions from the DHSS. Their plans to build a new laundry were vetoed, an intervention which forced the district to privatize the service.

But despite the interventionism from the centre the overall response of authorities to privatization was summed up by one commentator as a situation where 'Ministers [were] facing a mixture of rebellion and sullen procrastination from many health authorities' (*Guardian*, 13 June 1984).

Increasingly the issue of privatization indicated some of the fundamental debates around the organization of the NHS and in particular the role of management and the degree of autonomy of the districts. To study the progress of privatization is to facilitate a review of the relative impact of the economic as opposed to the political in decision-making in the NHS. It also is a good indicator of the paradoxical nature of the relationship between central government and the periphery.

Ostensibly one major rationale for privatization was to facilitate a withdrawal of the state from various areas of organisational life. It was a policy presented as an ideological commitment in the 1979 Conservative Party manifesto, was prominent in the election campaign of that year and had remained central to the rhetoric of policy-making since. It may be instructive to reflect on the presented rationale for policy in 1979. The view appeared clear; it was that the enlargement of the role of the state and a diminution of the role of the individual and of private enterprise had 'crippled the enterprise and effort on which a prosperous country with improving social services depended'. The United Kingdom's 'relative economic decline could be reversed by the government working with the grain of human nature, helping people to help themselves – and others' (Conservative Party 1979, pp. 6–7). In the field of health and welfare this philosophy was to find expression in an intention to limit the role of the state in direct service provision and of central government in the management of local services, whether statutory or non-statutory. The approach of DHSS ministers was to be characterized, in their central-local relations, by disengagement, a term used in a speech by the Parliamentary Under Secretary for Health, Sir George Young, in anticipating the likely relationship between central government and the health service in the 1980s (quoted in Webb and Wistow 1982, p. 31). The Secretary of State rejected the view that ministers should preside over every detailed policy decision and that everything should be managed from Whitehall, saying that 'It is the government's firm policy that detailed planning and management of resources are best left to those on the spot who know local needs and priorities' (DHSS Press Notice 80/201, 5 August 1980).

By 1984 we could see that policy in operation and observe the paradox of the need for a more interventionist state to implement 'disengagement'. Conservatism cannot embrace the free market model without increasing other areas of control – or else the fear would be that to give 'freedom' means that those you give it to may not exercise choice in the way you want them to.

In the privatization of hospital services by June 1984, ten authorities had decided not to comply with the directive to put services out to tender.

Twelve had decided to maintain wages and conditions of service of ancillary staff at NHS levels, so making it difficult for private contractors to reduce wages, cut costs and win contracts. Another 55 health authorities had taken no action in submitting timetables for privatization. This left 157 authorities which had complied, at least to the extent of submitting timetables. However, such a response rate is somewhat misleading – they may have submitted timetables but these may have been of an order that did not correspond with the government expectations. For example, all the district authorities in the Northern Region had made returns but only half of these intended to follow the government guidelines and complete the programme by 1986. Some offered plans to complete by 1989. Other authorities had responded with imaginative schemes. Oxford offered crash courses so that its own staff would be in a better position to compete in bidding with outside contractors.

When authorities had put out services to tender the private sector had been successful in the cleaning contracts. By mid-1984, of 15 such services put out to tender, 13 had been given to private contractors. Among laundry services private contractors had won eight out of the nine that had been decided. In catering the picture was different, with the first five successful contracts going to NHS staff. Some proposed privatizations seemed to receive little attention from the private sector. South Warwickshire tried to privatize its vehicles maintenance services and asked 54 firms to tender; 12 replied and only two were interested in tendering for the complete service. The contract remained in-house (*Guardian*, 13 June 1984).

Disputes over privatization continued throughout 1985 but without the media prominence of 1984. The preoccupation of the new year in this area of policy was directed towards private medicine, with the role of the market and the activities of doctors in the pursuit of private work being the central concern. The Comptroller and Auditor General, Sir Gordon Downey, refused, in April 1985, to approve the 1983–4 NHS accounts. This provided a major embarrassment for the DHSS. These accounts, he said, pinpointed serious weaknesses in the system for collecting private patients' fees. It was a weakness that had led to losses of about £10 million a year. His study took in only 37 of the 192 health districts; if the situation he found had been repeated nationally the total cost would have been more of the order of £50 million – or £60 million if you take Michael Meacher's reading of the implications of the report (*Guardian*, 27 April 1985).

Authorities had failed to comply with DHSS guidelines and did not have adequate procedures to control income from private patients and other non-NHS work. The BMA was quick to point to this and to seek to absolve its members from blame and certainly from any suggestion of fraud. Looking at the detail of the report, it is difficult to absolve doctors from responsibility. For example, in Wakefield evidence was uncovered of referral of a patient direct to an NHS hospital X-ray department as an NHS patient when she had previously attended consultants' rooms in a private capacity (extracts from the Comptroller and Auditor General's Audit Report (1985) quoted in the *New Statesman*, 10 May 1985, pp. 12–13). Certainly it is consultants who are the ones to gain from such practices. In May two consultant pathologists were suspended by West Midlands Regional Health Authority pending an investigation into irregularities identified in the Audit Report concerning collection of private fees. They were suspended on full pay and received assurances from the BMA that it would defend them if they were dismissed (*Guardian* 16 May 1985).

In June an 18-month inquiry by the House of Commons Public Accounts Committee (PAC) (House of Commons Committee of Public Accounts 1986c), Parliament's watchdog on government expenditure, reported on the study of profits amassed by the British Oxygen Company (BOC) from sales to the NHS. The inquiry had been stimulated by a joint investigation by the *Guardian* and the College of Health (a body set up in 1983 to act as a pressure group to push the interests of NHS patients and made up of, among others, doctors, professors, medical college presidents and consumer campaigners). BOC was a monopoly supplier of medical gases to the NHS and its contract was worth £16 million in 1983. It also was paid a further £16 million for medical equipment. The Report was complex and equivocal in assessing whether there had been excess charges. In itself it provided a fascinating example of the sorts of relationship that could exist between an inquiry, under the aegis of a Parliamentary committee, and the private sector. Some of the issues that came up, mainly in a minority report of the PAC (Minority Report 1986), provided glimpses of that area of commercial profit and the NHS where the power of private monopoly is considerable. While most publicity concentrates on private medicine and putting out to tender NHS work, it is in the long-standing relationship with the private sector for the supply of drugs and medical equipment that the power of private monopoly suppliers (protected by patent in the case of many drugs) remains considerable.

The government agreement with BOC had been negotiated and agreed using a rate that assessed the contract as high risk and so offered higher reimbursement. It is hard to understand why it should be high risk when one can safely anticipate that the NHS will continue to need oxygen and BOC will remain a monopoly supplier. The rate of return for BOC was estimated at 20.5 per cent in 1982, as against an average return for capital in industrial and commercial companies of 13.8 per cent that year. A Monopolies Commission report (House of Commons Trade and Industry Committee 1973; see also Monopolies and Restrictive Practices Commission 1957) had suggested that where companies were in a monopoly position they should achieve a rate of return lower than the industrial average. There was also concern that innovative new techniques for the domestic supply of oxygen were being proposed by the company in such a way as to preserve their monopoly of supply.

The whole tenor of the Report and the Minority Report that accompanied it was one of uncertainty about the relationship between the DHSS and this major private sector contractor (*Guardian*, 7 June 1985). But the majority report did not commit itself to specifics. One might conclude that the decision-making and planning procedures of the DHSS were not well equipped to operate in these matters. The response of the DHSS had been to appoint private management consultants (they appointed two firms to look at hospital medical gas prices and at the options available in providing a domestic medical gas service). This seems only to highlight the problems in keeping a detailed check on the private sector and to bode ill if there was a considerable expansion of private sector encroachment on service delivery in the NHS.

The developing relationship between the NHS and commercial interests included the NHS seeking some extra revenue by opening up facilities to private firms, commercialization rather than privatization – or, to use the words that typified the approach, 'a concern with revenue generation'. Hospitals were planning to rent space to retailers – florists, banks, fast food outlets, even undertakers – to open on hospital premises. Some schemes were begun quietly and were being slowly developed. In the main they appeared to be quietly successful and certainly contributed small amounts to income. There were some failures. At Addenbrooke's Hospital in Cambridge the introduction of a commercial photographer into the maternity ward did not work – the hospital administrator thought it might have been construed as too pushy! As well as the development of this sort of enterprise health authorities were considering opening private screening facilities and commercial sports clinics (*Guardian*, 26 September 1985).

The year 1985 saw the opening of a private, profit-making, psychiatric hospital for people compulsorily detained by the state. It was located in Cambridgeshire, run by American Medical International, and aimed to take patients from health authorities which did not have enough secure places themselves. It was to charge £690 a week per patient. Critics, including Tony Smyth, Secretary of the Association of Community Health Councils, saw this as the start of a move towards privatizing psychiatric hospitals and then prisons using an American model (*Guardian*, 9 October 1985).

Private hospitals were given the go-ahead to carry out liver transplant operations using organs donated through the NHS as long as there were no suitable NHS recipients or recipients in European countries who had reciprocal agreements with the United Kingdom. The charge for such an operation at the Cromwell Hospital, London, was between £25,000 and £35,000. One of the surgeons involved stressed that there were no suitable

NHS patients and that additionally the 'nationally funded programme at Addenbrooke's and King's is very stretched. It's sometimes easier to do transplants in a private hospital which is geared to looking after these patients. It helps to spread the load' (Dr Williams, Director of the Cromwell liver unit and head of the NHS liver research unit at King's College Hospital, London, quoted in the *Guardian*, 5 November 1985). During the year five private patients and 40 NHS patients had been given liver transplants.

Private health care insurance had seen a peak growth rate of 20 per cent a year fall to little more than 3 per cent a year in the five years up to 1985. The companies involved appeared to be responding in two ways. Either they increased premiums (BUPA imposed an 11 per cent rise from 1 January 1986) or they cut benefits and expanded exclusion clauses. This was the path taken by the second largest company, Private Patients Plan (PPP). Their new scheme would exclude long-term kidney dialysis, infertility treatment, drug abuse and alcoholism. Policy holders wanting cover for psychiatric treatment, pregnancy complications and out-patient services would have to pay an extra 15 per cent on their premium. Further, they would be offered the possibility of paying between £85 and £220 of the cost of treatment and so being eligible for further reduced premiums. Such changes did not please American Medical International (nor, one suspects, other private hospitals) which had recently expanded into alcohol, drug and psychiatric treatment. Its Managing Director called the decision narrow-minded and negative and he accused PPP of taking the easy way out. The move, he said, went against all the trends in the growing private health care sector where the direction of change was towards more comprehensive care (*Guardian*, 6 December 1985). It must have been music to the ears of some NHS workers and administrators to hear of the private sector's costs problem and the division within their ranks!

The profitability of private firms contracting and providing services to the NHS remained an issue throughout 1986. So did continuing discussion on the value of private hospital care and whether some of its costs were being met by the NHS because of uncharged fees. Indeed, there was a DHSS directive (DHSS 1986c) to appoint private patient officers to NHS hospitals to stop the loss of charges. The context of such concern was not just the Audit Report, described above, but the realization of how considerable the commitment of NHS doctors to the private health sector now was. A report from NHS Unlimited (1986) (a group formed to combat private medicine) showed that 50 health authorities had failed to collect money from private patients, or had allowed their facilities to be used by consultants without proper charges. As to involvement in private practice, the number of full-time consultants earning more than 10 per cent of their income from private practice in five health regions studied jumped from 95 to 295 in four years. In Peterborough alone 12 out of 38 doctors dropped their full-time commitment to the NHS within weeks of the opening of a new private hospital (*Guardian*, 11 March 1986).

A new method of preparing hospital food, called cook-chill, provoked a very interesting discussion that helps us understand some of the conflicting pressures in the NHS at this time. Cook-chill is a method of food preparation that was offered to the NHS by Gardner Merchant, the United Kingdom's largest private catering company and a subsidiary of Trusthouse Forte. It had not been involved in the initial round of competing for contracts to cater for the NHS. In fact the attempt to involve the private sector in this area had been largely unsuccessful; only seven out of the total of 2500 hospital contracts had gone to the private sector. What the company wanted was long-term contracts with health authorities which would not have been considered if only the lowest tender was acceptable. They planned a programme that would require substantial capital investment.

The thinking behind this approach was supported by the NHS Management Board and would be supported by many NHS managers. There was a general realization that the 'easy' cost cutting exercises had been done. Now if any substantial improvement was to be made it would have to include some capital spending. This, it was hoped, would be offset in the longer term by revenue saving, and would also lead to an improved service for patients and better conditions for staff. Cook-chill was not the only example; others include the installation of new telephone switchboards.

But the emphasis of the political agenda was different. It centred on a wish to speed up the process of tendering for cleaning, laundry, linen and catering services in hospitals. The Junior Health Minister, Ray Whitney, had been given six months to present substantial savings in the NHS regardless of whether contracts went to the private or the public sector. The emphasis now seemed to be on increasing the figure that could be claimed as total efficiency savings. Quick savings were the order of the day (*Guardian*, 12 March 1986). It was to be the presentation of policy that took precedence. The government wished to argue that its privatization policy was successful but also, and now more so, that it was 'more efficient' in its utilization of funds within the NHS. This was another area in which there was a contradiction between policy objectives and one in which the relative dominance of one over another changed over time and in response to calculations of political expediency.

Up to March 1986 the savings from competitive tendering in the NHS were identified by the government as being up to £52 million pounds a year. Since the privatization programme had begun 251 NHS contracts had been awarded to private contractors and 700 to in-house tenders. Two things were happening that would influence the picture on efficiency savings. First, a series of mergers and takeovers meant that among contract cleaning firms there were now near-monopoly conditions in some areas. Seven companies had been awarded 70 per cent of the contracts to supply domestic staff to the NHS and one of those, Hawley, had almost a third of the contracts awarded for domestics and cleaning. Second, as firms returned with renewed estimates after the completion of the initial contract these had been significantly higher. There was now no in-house team to compete against (*Guardian*, 30 September 1986).

Overall, the government was experiencing reverses in its attempts to reduce moneys paid out to the private sector. The drugs bill rose by £121 million in 1985, despite the introduction of the limited drugs list. That rise, which meant the drugs bill was £1786.6 million, represented a 7.3 per cent rise at a time when inflation was running at 5.6 per cent. There is a Pharmaceutical Price Regulation Scheme (PPRS) which is meant to decide on the profit levels drug companies can make. We were not allowed to know what profit levels were because the committee met in secret and the results of its negotiations were subject to the Official Secrets Act. The part of the DHSS that was involved with the drug companies appeared considerably underresourced. Thirteen people were supposed to scrutinize the balance sheets of the 60 international drug companies who supplied the NHS.

In 1983 the Secretary of State had made some figures in this area public when he announced a 2.5 per cent cut in NHS drug prices and a price freeze into the following year (DHSS 1983b). He subsequently (DHSS 1984c) said that the average profit target for the industry was being cut back from 25 per cent to 21 per cent, as measured by capital employed. In November 1984 he ordered a further cut to 17 per cent (at the same time as the limited list was introduced). Despite the anguished protests of the drug companies at every step the real dilemma was in knowing if the costs they claimed could be validated.

There appeared a widespread suspicion that practices such as transfer pricing, bogus research, encouragement of the introduction of needless drugs and the establishment of bogus competition were all devices used to cloak real costs and hence to hide the real profit margins allowed under government agreement (*Guardian*, 23 July 1986). Bogus research is that process whereby drug trials are introduced into various doctors' surgeries. They are really thinly disguised promotional exercises but are included in research costs and so used to justify higher prices and profits. Transfer pricing is where a drug company artificially inflates the cost of raw materials from a foreign subsidiary and in so doing falsely boosts declared costs and hence can achieve higher profits than those it appears to be getting through PPRS packages.

As if the situation was not favourable enough to the drug companies, in 1986 Norman Fowler announced new PPRS agreements which would allow a return, by 1987, to the notional profit target of 21 per cent. A long-term change was proposed whereby PPRS would be abandoned and drug industry profits linked, via the *Financial Times* 500 Index, to the performance of other companies. To facilitate a harmonious shift to the new arrangements 'sweeteners' were offered including possible increases in profit bonuses and increased allowances for promotional spending. The industry's journal welcomed these as a set of measures that would restore confidence and provide for a period of stability in the industry (*Guardian*, 19 August 1986). The government did appear to be making some attempt to come to terms with transfer pricing and to exclude capital spent on producing generic drugs from the pricing equations. But a government apparently intent on cost cutting and efficiency savings remained generous to a private industry which received a large proportion of NHS revenue and which had been reaping large profits from the sale of its products to the NHS.

The discussions over BOC and the pharmaceutical industry serve to remind us that in relations between the NHS and the private sector the danger is that an emphasis will be unduly placed on new privatization to the exclusion of the long-standing role of business enterprise. It is the level of profit this exacts and the lack of control exercised by the government that should be subject to close and continuing scrutiny. There appears potential for profit to be taken out of the NHS in such a way as to make the sorts of sums gained in efficiency savings exercises seem small. There is a peculiar myopia in which the excesses of private enterprise are overlooked while the small print of in-house work is studied for every saving and in which staff salaries are kept as low as possible. This is not just a feature of the NHS. It is reminiscent of the disproportionate attention paid, for example, to social security fraud as against the hugely more lucrative practice of tax evasion.

One area of problems for the NHS has been in realizing its no longer needed assets. In January 1987 there was considerable criticism of the sale of a former NHS psychiatric hospital in County Durham. The hospital was sold to a person who made an unsolicited private bid. It was not advertised (although it was valued by the District Valuer) and it was sold before the usual advice of the PAC that in such case planning permission should first be sought to enhance the value and hence price of the property and its land (*Guardian*, 6 January 1987: see also the *Guardian*, 9 January 1987).

By 1987 the situation in regard to competitive tendering was that savings to be accrued from it appeared to be diminishing, and some firms were losing interest in bidding for contracts. By the original target date for the completion of competitive tendering, September 1986, tenders had been invited on only 70 per cent of cleaning, catering and laundry services. Those contracts so far awarded were expected to generate annual savings of £73 million, which would amount to 20 per cent of previous costs. Private contractors had been awarded 55 per cent of tenders in the period from January 1984 to March 1985 but in the period from July to September 1986 they took only 8 per cent. The private sector had been most successful in winning cleaning contracts. Laundry and particularly catering remained in-house. Private bids have done much better in London and the Home Counties than the North, Scotland and Wales. In its study of tendering the Comptroller and Auditor General's office assessed, as the reason for the success of in-house bids, a combination of their being more ready to cut costs (they had certainly been prepared to renegotiate bonus schemes and to use a greater amount of part-time work than before), and an unpreparedness on the part of the private sector to enable them to match the pace and scale of the tendering exercise. 'The tendering initiative was seen by one Commons Committee as having proved a much needed spur towards improved efficiency although more work might be needed' (National Audit Office 1987). One might surmise that a spur towards accepting worse working arrangements was the pool of unemployed and the ever present risk to the jobs of NHS workers from the tender process. The other features absent from the calculation about profit and loss were the quality of service offered and the long-term impact on the health and morale of staff.

Health authorities had 'insured' themselves by the use of performance bonds which indemnified authorities if contractors failed to meet their work targets. But the NHS Management Board advised against the continued use of such bonds on the grounds that they were unnecessary if the health authorities carried out proper vetting when examining contractors and tenders (*Guardian*, 4 February 1987). We might remember the Cornish experience of being overruled by the Ministry when they thought they had done their vetting.

If savings from this round of competitive tendering and privatization were limited this did not deter the government from seeking new areas. In the time-honoured way some possibilities were floated to test opinion and then rejected as being politically inexpedient – thus pathology laboratories and nurses' homes avoided being put out to tender. But apparently less sensitive areas that might be developed included hospital transport, sterile supplies, gardening, building, engineering, energy maintenance, and portering (*Guardian*, 22 May 1987).

Health Policy and the Politics of the 1980s

In this chapter I will look at those items of debate concerning the NHS, its functioning and development, which are not strictly included in considerations of detailed planning and management issues and which are not simply about expenditure levels or about the role of the private sector. Inevitably, however, these categories overlap. I want to consider some of the general questions about the sort of health service there should be and how it should link with the rest of society, and to look at how this was presented in the public debate of the years studied. This presentation concludes with an examination of issues of health policy as they were evident in the general election campaign of 1987. In seeking these general issues one comes across the idea that the health service sought was a better-managed, more efficient, cheaper and less centrally organized service and so what follows must be considered alongside previous chapters.

The year 1984 was one of agenda setting and the two main issues, for the government at least, were, first, the role of the NHS within a general economic strategy that was seeking to reduce public expenditure and, second, the sort of NHS they should be seeking. It appeared that the government were interested in looking at both the scale and the scope of the NHS it was to administer. The Labour Party and many other groups, including trade unionists and doctors, appeared to be setting longer-term objectives and considering the future. Their stance was if the first agenda was to defend the NHS this must be accompanied by a strategy that recognized its shortcomings and could prepare a policy of reform to overcome them.

One addition to the information on planning was that in 1984 the Public Expenditure White Paper (DHSS 1984b) contained details of spending for the next fiscal year as well as plans for 1985–6 and 1986–7. If the intention was admirable, to extend the amount of information available, the actuality was far from illuminating about anything other than the manipulability of figures. The White Paper came out in February and the revenue details were not announced until March. The excess of spending over revenue is the public sector borrowing requirement and it was this that the government was intent on reducing. The White Paper showed that this intention was not being realized. In fact the increase in public expenditure was to be of the order of 6.1 per cent (up to £120.328 billion) and this was 1 per cent above inflation.

The 'real' increase was more like 7 per cent but was not presented as such because the sell-off of nationalized assets was used to offset the figure. Counting asset sales as a reduction in expenditure is a dubious practice for two main reasons: first, it is not a long-term practical possibility (although the Chancellor did seem to see the possibilities of asset sales each year well into the 1990s); second, it hides the true picture of the way the public sector is developing *vis-à-vis* the whole economy. The government appeared to hope that public spending would reduce, national income grow and the result would leave room for tax cuts.

Even within such policy constraints there were a number of possibilities for the welfare state and for the NHS in particular. Theoretically it could be decided that even if public spending were to be controlled the amount given to the NHS would increase. But there are limitations on the government's freedom of action that are created by two types of consideration, economic and ideological.

Spending on unemployment benefits would cost 166 per cent of their 1978–9 levels without any one of the unemployed getting any more than before. Also high interest rates meant that debt interest would be 90 per cent higher, in real terms, than at the beginning of the 1980s. In the allocation of money among departments there was evident a continuing trend towards favouring the defence and law and order budgets over education, housing and health. This trend had been present in each White Paper on expenditure since 1979. By 1985 the increase in defence spending since 1979 was 27 per cent in real terms, the biggest peacetime expansion of modern times.

With all these calls on expenditure and a general policy to reduce it there should be no surprise that some departments do very badly both absolutely and relatively. In 1979 the health and personal social services budget was almost identical to that of defence – only £72 million less than defence's £7497 million. By 1985 the gap in money terms was £1610 million. The hardest hit department had been housing. If it is compared with law and order the change is dramatic. In 1979 the housing budget was almost twice that of law and order. By 1985 the positions were reversed; the housing budget was £2264 million and law and order £4446 million (1982 prices). Housing spending would be only one-third the amount the Conservative government had spent on it in its first year in office. Education had also been cut in real terms and social security had had more than £1500 million cut from its benefits. But the social security budget had increased because of the increase in unemployment, the number of one-parent families and the number of elderly.

Health spending had increased relative to education. Whereas in 1979 more had been spent on the latter than on health and personal social services, by 1985 not only were the positions reversed but the gap was more than £2000 million. The health and personal social services budget totalled £13,987 million (1982 prices).

The published estimates for future years indicated spending in cash terms rising by 5 per cent in 1984–5, by 4.5 per cent in 1985–6 and by 3.5 per cent in 1986–7, although the detailed distribution of these sums was not presented in the White Paper. It was expected that spending on health and social services would rise by 1.2 per cent in real terms in the financial year 1984–5 and then decline slightly in 1985–6. The figures were below even the most cautious estimate of what the NHS would have to receive to stay the same (DHSS 1984b; see also the *Guardian*, 17 February 1984).

Further, the assumptions about spending levels and the types of service that could be provided were based on a calculation about the rate of inflation that past experience suggested could not be so accurately predicted. Between 1979 and 1982 government plans had been considerably disrupted because the level of inflation was above that calculated for. Between 1982 and 1984 inflation was lower than expected and hence the government's plan looked much more successful. It is one of those phenomena that is not within the absolute control of a single government and can be seriously affected by a wide range of events. It is also one of those things that governments take credit for if the rate is low and disown as nothing to do with them if things go badly! To base a planning system on it is a considerable arrogance and it certainly means that any long-term planning must be very tentative and speculative.

These were the financial assumptions that the development of policy rested on. Some of the doctrine underpinning them became evident in the keynote speech the Prime Minister made to the Conservative Party Conference in October 1983. The NHS is not free, she reminded her supporters; in 1983 it had cost over £15 billion, a figure equal to half of all income tax. It had a million employees and was the largest employer in Europe. She identified the government's responsibility as being to see that such a huge undertaking was managed properly. Within that, she said, she rejected the socialist view that the most efficient organization was the one that employed the most people. The budget was huge and was growing but good management meant keeping within that budget. There was not a bottomless purse, the sky was not the limit and hard choices needed to be made. (There is nothing like reading the transcripts of politicians' speeches for collecting lists of cliches – it is not just the preserve of Mrs Thatcher!)

The figures she used were that £700 million more would be spent on health in 1983, £800 million in 1984, and a further £700 million in 1985. She concluded this part of her speech with a subsequently much-quoted attack on the Opposition, saying that it would spend, spend and spend before it had even filled in the coupon, let alone won the pools. As for the Conservatives, she reminded her audience that

> At this conference last year . . . I said 'The NHS is safe with us'. I will go further. The NHS is safe only with us because this government will see that it is prudently managed and financed, that care is concentrated on the patient rather than the bureaucrat. That is the true, the genuine care (Conservative Party Conference, 14 October 1983).

She compared the success of the NHS under the Conservatives with the problems experienced in other countries – boarding charges for hospital patients in socialist France, and cuts or indexing of social security in West Germany, the Netherlands, Belgium and Denmark.

It was a speech that was interpreted as identifying the government's clear commitment to the NHS. But it left that commitment dependent upon the broader success of economic policy. Its use of statistics was selective – to talk about increased amounts to be spent rather than about percentage increases makes it appear that large sums are generously being given whereas in reality the increase is small. Her European examples were well picked – on a number of other items the UK would not have compared so favourably.

Within the Labour Party the prospect of several more years in opposition had led, by 1984, to a shift from a preoccupation with trying to stop hospital closure and job cuts to a consideration of the wider issues of democracy in the NHS and its future organization and funding. The party seemed concerned to assess the types of service that would effectively respond to need in the conditions likely to be prevalent in the 1980s and 1990s. Such a rethink was closely associated with Michael Meacher, Labour's health spokesman. He also identified the state of the national economy, as opposed to the structure of the NHS, as being the single most important issue. In a speech in Oxford he seemed to acknowledge that the Labour Party, had it been in government, would probably have followed policies of restricting expenditure on the NHS similar to those of the Conservatives. But now he was seeking to both broaden the definition of health and health need to include a consideration of the consequences of growth and wealth. We must reappraise, he said, the whole question of the sort of growth we want. The economy ought to be a health-promoting economy (quoted in Rentoul and Cohen 1984). One interesting figure available to him was the findings of an economic, social and policy audit of the NHS (CIPFA 1984) which, as part of a comprehensive review, costed the output lost through illness and injury in the economy as a whole as £40 billion in 1981.

It is important for the Labour Party to own up to that part of its past that had seen it, in government, acting in ways similar to those it was now criticizing in the Conservatives. If it seeks to take advantage of the claim that it gave the United Kingdom the NHS then it must acknowledge the faults built into it from the outset and the subsequent record of underfunding and the submergence of the needs of health to the over-riding considerations of economic management. The dilemma for many in 1984 was whether that commitment to reappraisal was the Labour Party's or just Michael Meacher's.

The shift in priorities for NHS campaigners seemed to arise out of a realization of the absurdities of supporting the continued existence of outdated and unneeded facilities. London Health Emergency co-ordinator, Lucy de Groot, summed up the spirit of this change:

> The experience of anti-cuts campaigns in the 1970s showed a lot of activists that it is not enough to defend bits of the service that are there. These may be impersonal and not relevant to people's needs. When you find yourself defending an 1880s workhouse you have to start thinking: 'What is this all about' (quoted in Rentoul and Cohen 1984).

New preoccupations were about the need to develop more preventive medicine, the development of democracy within the NHS and a continuing concern with the impact of privatization.

The 'Who Cares' campaign, set up by ten trade unions in the Oxford region, provided an example of such a changed approach. It sought to campaign for a change in health priorities and to develop democratization in the NHS (Who Cares, c/o ASTMS Office, 18 St Clements, Oxford). Similar concerns were evident in the 'Strategy for Health' meetings which centred on Sheffield, ventured into Leeds and Bradford, and attracted people from all over Britain (Progressive Strategies for Health, c/o Central Policy Unit, Town Hall, Sheffield).

The year 1985 began with the publication of extracts of the annual report of the Health Service in 1984 (DHSS 1984a). All the indexes presented displayed unrelenting progress. It was a picture of a triumphant NHS tempered only by sober and level-minded consideration of the responsibilities and challenges of the future. Just before the Conservative Party Conference another leaflet (Health Circular (85)5) appeared similarly presenting the NHS as being in its best shape ever. In this leaflet the Secretary of State used patient attendance and out-patient appointments as an indication of the record level of service. He did not identify how many of these attendances were the same patient making repeated visits, perhaps because the first visit was not satisfactory. Nor did he consider the paradox that the figures may just indicate record levels of ill health existing in contemporary Britain. Among the other selective statistics was one of 24 new hospitals built since 1979 and 250 being planned, designed or built. No figure was given for how many hospitals had been closed. This leaflet, and the Annual Report, allowed the Secretary of State to arrive triumphant at the Party Conference. But his main focus during the year was not specifically on the NHS as such but on the proposals for a reform of the whole social security system.

Norman Fowler introduced a three volume Green Paper (DHSS 1985) which he billed as the most substantial examination of the social security system since the Beveridge Report. At the heart of the paper there appeared to be an intention by the Treasury and the Cabinet to effect a major reduction in the social security budget to aid the over-riding government imperative of a reduction in the public sector borrowing requirement. Fowler's problems centred on the likely long-term effect of the State Earnings Related Pensions (SERPS) and on child benefit. Both were paid irrespective of need and both served as a target for the government. The government aspired to shift the focus towards benefits paid according to need (as defined by itself, of course). Need could be defined according to the imperatives of economic policy and a measure of enhanced executive power achieved. The resulting long-running debate was, of course, central in a consideration of health policy because of the link between poverty, financial uncertainty and health. But it also was of importance in terms of seeking to identify the amount of funding that might specifically be available for the NHS.

The overall financial position of the NHS remained one in which there was some small increase in the absolute level of funding but that central to the Treasury's calculations was the expectation that funds for growth would be obtained by redirecting money from efficiency savings. The Chancellor's Autumn Financial Statement indicated that the government would increase the amount allocated to the NHS by £250 million in the financial year 1986–7. Almost half this sum would be needed to pay the staged pay award to doctors and nurses. The rest seemed to indicate a recognition of the increasing demands being made on services. But the amount allocated in itself was not enough to keep pace with such changes. The Chancellor's expectation was, however, that health authorities could make available a further £150 million by reorganizing services, including the closure of hospitals (*Guardian*, 13 November 1985).

In 1986 the suspended consultant, Wendy Savage, was reinstated and a new Junior Minister of Health, Edwina Currie, told northerners that their relative ill health was due in part to their own ignorance compared with the more enlightened southerners. In this year also there was a continuation of the general policy trends evident from preceding years. If there was a great deal of discussion about the NHS essentially there was a considerable degree of continuity, a lack of change, beneath the sound and fury.

This continuity in itself brought problems and early in 1986 a number of these were drawn to public attention when Professor Shuster, Professor of Dermatology at the University of Newcastle-upon-Tyne, pointed to the cumulative effect of cuts. The medical division of the teaching hospital in which he worked requested £250,000 for the replacement of essential equipment and got £19,000. This was a similar response to that of the previous year. The fabric and the resources of the hospital were being eroded and the level of spending required to bring them to a desirable state again did not appear forthcoming. Even using the government's good housekeeping homilies this was a dubious practice, he argued – who would not consider it sensible to replace the odd tile on the roof as it worked loose rather than saving the money and waiting until a gale brought the whole thing down?

Shuster also spoke of the bad housekeeping which a preoccupation with the budget of particular parts of the NHS produces. The hospital was told to reduce spending by £1 million. One thing it did was to stop dispensing for out-patients – they would have to go back to their GPs for prescriptions. Such a practice does mean the hospital can offset some spending but the total call on the NHS goes up as drugs obtained from the hospital, which can buy in bulk, are cheaper.

Further, cuts expressed as a percentage of total cost do not provide a picture of how they affect some parts of the hospital. Certain areas of specialism are more protected than others. If the long-term strategy is of developing services for the mentally ill, for example, then the percentage cuts have to be greater in areas like acute services. This may mean, in order to get the cuts required, closing whole units or whole wards irrespective of the degree of need. In Newcastle one suggestion was the closure of one of the two dermatology wards. If this were done it would leave the number of beds available for the treatment of skin disease at half the national norm (*Guardian*, 19 March 1986).

Michael Meacher's attempts to redraw Labour's health policy involved a series of study groups looking at different aspects of health care. Their suggestions were becoming public by 1986. Some of these were far-reaching, impressive, and were designed to redefine the understanding of what a policy for health could and should achieve. They were concerned to locate health in the overall context of social divisions and social change and to suggest that a policy for health would appear very different than the usual consensus on a policy for the treatment of illness. Some of the highspots of the report, called 'A New Vision for Health', included laws to stamp out smoking among all but the most hardened addicts; the direct election of health authorities to end what Meacher himself described as the existing system of political patronage and centralization of power that had grossly distorted the NHS over the previous seven years; the introduction of a health committee of ministers and Civil Servants to ensure that health needs are taken into account when other departments formulate policy; and finally – centrally – the recognition that bad housing, unemployment and shortcomings in public transport are central producers of ill health and need to be tackled as priorities in any health policy (*Guardian*, 28 May 1986).

This was the centrepiece report but others, prepared by policy advisory teams, also reported to Michael Meacher. One recommended that the drugs bill could be controlled by buying a drug firm for the nation. Such a step, it was envisaged, would be achieved by buying a 51 per cent share on the stock market. The firm would generate profits and compete with the private sector. In so doing it would hopefully contribute to a decline in prices charged to the NHS. Further, it would allow its new owners access to the books and hence give them an insight into the PPRS and the scale of profits this firm, and presumably others, had been really obtaining from the NHS (*Guardian*, 21 May 1986).

These reports were symptomatic not just of the lasting malaise and the need for drastic action that many workers and users of the NHS were experiencing by 1986 but also of a recognition of the shortcomings of a policy line built around just defending what already exists and promising more of the same. Developing such critiques is typical of the Labour Party in opposition when an election is not close and is transformed into a more narrow instrumentality in aims and conventionality in aspiration when manifestos come to be written.

Outside the Labour Party study groups the debate during 1986 was still dominated by contradictory claims about figures. Each year the report of the House of Commons Social Services Select Committee provided a clearing ground for the examination of health service spending and the scale of provision as compared to need. I have gone over the arguments often in the preceding pages; certainly in 1986 the points made remained the same. The government claimed to be spending more money and treating more patients than ever before. Scrutiny of the figures led to two kinds of criticism. One was that the first point might be true but more was not enough to compensate for a rate of price inflation in items central to the NHS that exceeded the national average. Wage costs rising faster than inflation were one feature of this, as were rises in drug and equipment prices. Nor was it enough to compensate for demographic changes or the need to keep up with new technology.

The second line of argument was that the figures themselves were misleading. They no longer compared like with like – the government had changed what a patient was (it was an admission and not a body) and changed what a nurse was (it was a number of hours worked and not an employee). It had also redistributed, via RAWP, the way money was allocated which had left some areas, notably in the South-East, with absolute reductions in funding levels and hence with 'real cuts'. They talked of efficiency savings as money for growth and confused the discussion on health budgets by sometimes including GP funds and hospital funds in the same presentations. This prevented the possibility of comparison between one year's set of figures and another (House of Commons Social Services Committee 1986).

But these arguments had been joined so many times before that what is perhaps of most importance is to understand them as a dominant discursive formation. It was the fact that such things were again being said rather than the specifics of detail that was crucial. From such an understanding one can seek the nature of communication and its role in shaping what is perceived as possible. To repeat the same assertions and hear the same rebuttals endlessly does suggest that the interchanges are not to be understood as rational dialogue concerned with advancing knowledge!

A further complication in assessing the state of the NHS was the need to evaluate the impact of the growth of private medicine. The private sector had expanded at a very considerable rate. In 1976, when the Labour government started to try and phase out private beds in NHS hospitals, there were 4900 pay beds in the NHS and 3500 in private hospitals. By 1986 there were 3500 pay beds in the NHS and 10,000 in private hospitals. Two consultants were quoted in a newspaper article (*Observer*, 18 May 1986) which identified the harmful impact on the NHS of the growth of the private sector. Professor Sam Shuster spoke of private medicine as parasitic, creaming off the relatively easy work, what he called 'cold surgery', non-urgent cases, and leaving the NHS with emergencies, most cancer and transplant surgery and the treatment of chronic complaints. Further, he said, the NHS was likely to get patients for whom things go wrong while they are being treated in the private sector. Mr Sam Galbraith, then a consultant neurosurgeon in Glasgow (now a Labour MP), concentrated on the moonlighting that goes on in the NHS and offered the following scenario for comparison. Imagine, he said, that British Airways allowed its pilots to work simultaneously for British Midland Airways. Furthermore, that these pilots could please themselves as to when, and if, they turned up for work. You arrive at Heathrow to catch the shuttle for Glasgow. Unfortunately there is no flight; the pilot has just taken off to Paris with British Midland and more than likely he has taken the British Airways plane with him. 'In the NHS highly paid hospital consultants are allowed, in the company's time and often using the company's equipment, to run what is in effect a rival business.' These are the complaints of just two critics of private health, but, as Sir Douglas Black, former president of the Royal College of Physicians, said: 'At every hospital one knows there are one or two doctors skimping on their public work for the sake of their private patients.'

The government, which prioritized presentation, was by mid-1986 becoming increasingly concerned with the vulnerability of its image as protector of the NHS (it anticipated an election in the coming year). So it mounted a counter-attack, with the Secretary of State, his ministers and the DHSS taking on the all-party House of Commons Social Services Committee's (1986) criticisms of the performance of the NHS.

DHSS (1986a) suggested that the Committee did not understand the figures and the nature of the government's commitment *vis-à-vis* funding. The Committee had criticized the government for only half doing what it had committed itself to do – to increase funding at a rate commensurate with need, given the generally accepted figure of 2 per cent necessary to compensate for demographic and specific cost increases. The DHSS pointed to 'the ultimate test [lying] not in any artificial and theoretical comparison between inputs [the 2 per cent figure] but what has actually happened to output – i.e. services provided and policy aims met'. The Committee, said the DHSS, had ignored the contribution of efficiency savings and improved productivity.

The government was committed to taking action to reduce waiting lists, a pledge made at the Conservative Party Conference by the Secretary of State who, in a rare display of flamboyance, had brandished a long list of planned hospital building projects. He offered the hope that by 1990 the number of heart bypass operations would increase from 7000 to 17,000, hip operations from 12,000 to 50,000, and cataract operations from 15,000 to 70,000 a year. Further, bone marrow transplants would be increased to at least 550 a year and cervical cancer screening supported by a call and recall system and by a speeding-up of the receipt of results. Finally, by the end of 1988 no mentally handicapped child receiving long-term care should be required to live in a large mental handicap hospital (*Guardian*, 9 October 1986).

Given the DHSS's wish to be judged by results it would, one can guess, not have been happy about the publication of the report from the Office of Population Censuses and Surveys (OPCS 1986). This report identified the health gap between the rich and poor as having grown sharply in the first four years of Conservative government after 1979. Death rates among young semi-skilled and unskilled workers aged 25–44 were more than twice as high as those for professional men and managers of the same age. Women married to men in social classes four and five were up to 70 per cent more likely to die young than wives of men in classes one and two (this is unfortunately how the figures are presented – they identify women as appendages of men!).

The results were a clear indication of the way death and disease had risen and would continue to rise along with poverty and unemployment. Compared with the rich, the poor were getting sicker and dying younger. Comparing the death rate for men in social classes four and five with that for men in social classes one and two in 1972 and then comparing the same groups in 1982 showed that the excess of the former over the latter groups had grown from 90 per cent to a 120 per cent. Prior to this period the level of inequality remained relatively stable for men over a 60-year period (see Townsend and Davidson 1982; and N. Hart, quoted in the *Guardian*, 30 July 1986).

For married women the entire post-war period had been one of steadily increasing inequality. Between 1972 and 1982 the difference in the risk of dying before retirement between the top and bottom social groups increased by 14 per cent for women. The trend had begun before the election of the Conservative government and, as such, the figures act as an indictment of the performance of the previous Labour government as well as of the post-1979 government.

Apart from the actual information presented in the OPCS (1986) report, the nature of its publication would support an argument that the government was embarrassed by its findings. For the first time since 1911 the crucial detailed analysis of deaths in different social classes had been omitted from the main report. They were contained in tables printed on microfiche and so available only to those people with the special facilities for looking at them, and they cost £40 to buy. The report had been finished at the beginning of 1986 but was not made available until July, four days after the Commons summer recess began. (This serves as a reminder about the similar treatment of the Black Report (Townsend and Davidson 1982) and about the manoeuvres engaged in by the Health Education Council to get its reports published and disseminated, as described on pages 60 and 61).

The bad news for a government which 'wished to be judged by results' continued into 1987 with the publication of a detailed report (Nutbeam and Catford 1987) based on a survey carried out on 22,000 people in Wales by the government-backed project to prevent heart disease and strokes, Heartbeat, Wales. One of its findings was the not surprising observation that the health gap between those in work and the unemployed was widening. The Welsh survey reinforced the findings of the Office of Population Censuses and Surveys. It added to it detailed findings on type of illness and linked these with occupational groupings. Those in manual groups, for example, were 32 per cent more likely to die of heart attacks and strokes than non-manual groups. It was a widening gap. Manual groups were two to three times as likely to display symptoms of angina, breathlessness and persistent coughs (the unemployed fared even more badly). Manual groups and the unemployed believed they had less control over their ability to reduce the risks of heart attack. 'This suggests that there is increased fatalism amongst these groups and may help to explain why unhealthy lifestyles are more common.'

Unhealthy lifestyles are then itemized around diet, weight, smoking and alcohol use. Manual groups ate more foods high in saturated fat, such as chips and processed meats, and fewer polyunsaturated margarines and vegetables. The unemployed had, in general, the poorest diet. The lower the social class the more likely people were to be overweight or obese. Over 7 per cent of women in social class five were dangerously obese as compared to 1 per cent in social class one. Nearly half the people in social class five smoked compared with under a quarter in class one. The unemployed smoked most of all. More unemployed men drank to excess: 9 per cent drank dangerously, compared with 8.5 per cent of men in class five and 4.5 per cent of men in class one (*Guardian*, 20 February 1987).

As I have indicated above, another study which reported on the widening gap between the health of the rich and poor, that of the Health Education Council (1987), came out in March. Its appearance was surrounded by controversy. Only 2000 copies were printed at first printing and a press conference planned for its launch was cancelled. Not even everyone in the House of Lords who wanted one could obtain a copy. The Lords were debating the NHS just after the report came out and the government was criticized for appearing to suppress yet another report critical of its performance in health. That debate did allow the Junior Health Minister, Baroness Trumpington, to respond to some of the recent criticisms. She told their Lordships that

> health differences among different groups in our society are of long standing. They have been a feature of life under [both Labour and Conservative] governments . . . a good diet and a healthy lifestyle do not depend on a high income . . . drinking and smoking . . . cost money . . . Overall, health in the United Kingdom has improved steadily. Life expectancy continues to rise. Infant mortality has fallen by one-third since 1979. [Improvements like these] reflect the increased resources [the government has] put into the health service, from £7.75 billion in 1978–1979 to nearly £20 billion next year (House of Lords, Parliamentary Debates, 30 March 1987, vol. 486, cols 356–60).

All of the debates that link health with aspects of individual behaviour and that assume the importance of choice have to be tempered by being located within a structural critique of contemporary society. It is perhaps progress to link unhealthy behaviour with the sense of futility and absence of power over one's life that is the result of poverty and, more particularly, of unemployment. But to pathologize in this way is to ignore two factors. The first is that the message about what constitutes a healthy lifestyle is not one that is always clearly communicated. It is countered by the mis-information of interested parties who want to persuade us that their product is good for us. Or the publicity is couched in such a way as to appeal differentially to groups from higher social classes. Second, the options for a healthy lifestyle may not be present. To live on a housing estate on the fringe of town, with an inadequate and expensive bus service, will mean that access to shops is limited. The estate shop's choice may not include those items conducive to healthy eating (the problem of trying to buy a wholemeal loaf on a housing estate may be something of a cliché, but *you* try it!). Such restrictions on choice are compounded by a shortage of money which means that items have often to be bought just a few at a time and in small quantities.

The series of reports that linked health and poverty, identifying a worsening of inequalities in health, had not ended. The BMA Board of Science was in the latter stages of completing a report, early drafts of which indicated a considerable agreement with the findings of the Health Education Council (1987) report. The report was to conclude by saying that

> In the interests of both justice and public health there should be a national commitment to combat social inequalities and eliminate deprivation... We call for a stronger political will to bring about changes in the deeply stratified nature of British society (*Guardian*, 28 March 1987).

The other report that addressed some of the same issues was being prepared on child health for the Health Education Council and the National Children's Bureau (National Children's Bureau 1987). This identified an increase in the number of children living in poverty and was critical of an absence of any increase in health checks, care or facilities to respond to what was an identifiable increase in need. The report sought to monitor improvements and changes in the development of an integrated service for children, of the sort recommended by the Court Report (DHSS 1976b) of ten years earlier, that would see children through their pre-school and school years. The Court Report had not been implemented. Adequate funds had not been provided nor had appropriate staff been appointed. Death rates among babies of unskilled workers were twice as high as those among babies born to parents in the professions (*Guardian*, 17 June 1987). The new report recommended that at least one paediatrician with special interest in community child care should be appointed in each health district. Second, efficient planning procedures should be established to ensure that the disparate parts of the NHS worked effectively together. The continuing difficulties of developing a unified service was attributed to the long-standing problems of co-operation within a fundamentally divided NHS.

The report also proposed adding to the health funding equation a 'poverty supplement' to enable the NHS to maintain its services. It was no longer enough just to add on the demographic and inflationary figures, agreed by all parties concerned; this additional identifiable increase in need ought to be funded.

As an interesting postscript to this debate a report from the National Perinatal Epidemiology Unit (Campbell and Macfarlane 1987) was critical of the policy of successive governments in encouraging women to give birth in hospital rather than at home. Home births had fallen from 19,000 in 1975 to less than 6000 in 1985. Almost all the 660,000 babies born in 1985 were born in hospital and the vast majority, 630,000, in consultant-staffed units at district hospitals. Perinatal mortality rates, babies born dead or dying soon after birth, had dropped from 19.2 per 1000 in 1975 to 9.8 per 1000 in 1985. The mortality rates for babies delivered at home was more than twice that for hospital births. But the home birth figures were considerably worsened by the proportion of deaths that occurred in unplanned home deliveries. When there had been plans, supported by the community services, the rate was 4.5 per 1000. In other words it may, with proper planning and the provision of the proper back-up facilities, be safer to have your baby at home.

Such research findings need careful scrutiny to identify causal factors in perinatal mortality. Perhaps all the more difficult cases are in hospital anyway and so the rate of problems would be higher than the planned home delivery rate. But the research does suggest the need to scrutinize common and accepted 'wisdom' within the medical profession. Certainly planners should consider the provision of a much wider range of choice as to where babies can be born, from high-technology specialist-led units, through 'cottage hospital' GP units, to a properly supported home delivery service.

Also likely to be received as bad news by the government was the consensus of opinion in reports that the dominant pressures upon the NHS were likely to demand an ever increasing health budget. In these circumstances a debate was gaining momentum as to alternate ways of allocating finance to different specialisms and to different forms of treatment. The dominant practice in deciding much of the allocation of a health authority's budget had been an annual round of bidding by consultants. 'Often it is decided on a basis of emotion and shroud waving' (Teeling-Smith 1987). I have looked at the suggestion that treatments should be justified using a basis of comparing cost with an assessment of how a patient feels and functions after treatment (the 'Quality Adjusted Life Year'). As well as the value of debating this and any other schemes, the observations about child birth above do underline the shortsightedness of any cut in research effort to evaluate the comparative benefit of treatments and to question long-standing, but not research-validated, assumptions about correct practice.

One suggestion to change the process by which money was allocated within health authorities involved the introduction of clinical budgets for doctors. Different health districts, and indeed different consultants within the same district, used more resources than others for treating the same condition. The Royal College of Physicians said that doctors had to accept management while ensuring that it operated in ways with which they were agreed. They proposed holding a series of seminars for consultants on financial management within the NHS and a parallel series for non-medical health managers to discuss the relative value of different options for clinical investigation and treatment. Sir Raymond Hoffenberg, President of the Royal College, put it thus:

> No country can do all of the things that are possible for all patients all of the time, so decisions on rationing or resource allocation have to be made ... these choices are now becoming more exposed and the college has taken a policy decision to urge doctors to be fully involved.

Dr Wickings of the King's Fund believed that clinical budgeting could be the only way to improve NHS care within Treasury spending limits. The aim should be, he said, to provide more or better care at the same cost rather than put doctors under managerial control (*Guardian*, 21 May 1987).

A report from three leading professional organizations – the Institute of Health Service Management (representing NHS staff), the BMA and the Royal College of Nursing (O'Higgins 1987) – proposed that spending on health should rise at least in line with growth in national income and should have additional provision to cope with population changes and with new areas of concern, such as the response to AIDS. If such a basis of resource allocation had been implemented in 1987–8 it would have meant an extra £172 million being spent, a 3.8 per cent rise in real NHS spending as opposed to the 2.8 per cent the government expected. But a much bigger gap would exist in 1988–9, when government projections were of 0.8 per cent and so the resulting deficit over the spending target proposed by these three organizations would be £600 million. This would rise to £900 million in 1989–90.

These higher spending figures, it was argued, would correspond to the rate of economic growth which appeared destined to pull away from the level of expenditure on the NHS if the advised course of action was not implemented. O'Higgins assumed that efficiency savings would continue at an annual saving of between 0.5 and 1 per cent of total budgets but argued that such savings should be kept within the service for funding real improvements and not used as a means of facilitating less government spending. It also identified that even the figures it suggested did not include sufficient for a programme of capital renewal. The deteriorating state of NHS plant would become a major issue in the kinds of service that could be provided and in the costs of upkeep and renewal that would become essential.

These reports identified a paradox in funding policy. We have made the assumption throughout that increased spending on the NHS has been dependent on the rate of growth in the national economy. By 1987 the centrepiece of government rhetoric was the claim that the United Kingdom had entered a period of sustained, and real, growth. But these reports argued that the allocation of funds to the NHS did not reflect that claimed economic reality. There has never been a straightforward link between the operation of the economy and the level of health funding. It is mediated by the exigencies of pressure group politics, is considered in a competitive arena and above all reflects estimates of political expediency. The new component now is an economic orthodoxy that attributes government expenditure as being an inhibitor to the progression of economic growth. The result is to replace a positive with a negative connection – previously it might have been argued that we can now afford to spend more on the welfare state because the economy is doing well. Now it is argued that the economy is doing well because we have been successful in limiting government spending. So increased health spending becomes a threat to economic growth.

To offer a point of focus at the end of this review of events in health policy as they have been identified in the public sphere I will look at the arguments around health and the NHS as they featured in the 1987 general election.

The party manifestos all featured health as a subject worthy of concern, of course. The Conservatives, in *The Next Moves Forward* (Conservative Party 1987) appealed for support on the basis of their record in office. We have seen how they had been seeking to present themselves as the only real defenders of the NHS. They claimed to have increased funding and introduced sound management.

But the manifesto was not detailed in its proposals of things to come. It did offer 125 new hospital building schemes in three years and spoke of more cervical and breast cancer screening. Preventive medicine would be supported through the new Health Education Authority and there would be monitoring of the community care policy and the management efficiency of the NHS. But essentially it subsumed health policy under the more general considerations described above and health was identified more as an issue in speeches than in the manifesto.

The Labour Party had engaged in the very interesting detailed examination of policy described on pages 107–8. This included many challenges to the orthodoxies practised in health planning and decision-making by earlier governments of both parties. But the manifesto, titled *Britain Will Win* (Labour Party 1987) did not reflect this. Labour's proudest achievement, it said, was the NHS. It offered cuts in hospital waiting lists through computerized bed allocation, more local health centres and well woman clinics and more money for AIDS research. Prescription charges would be reduced and eventually abolished and there would be a phasing out of pay beds and a removal of public subsidies to private health. Privatization in the NHS would be ended.

This was a very conventional programme and in substance, if not in detail, could have been produced at any time since the 1950s. The detail – computers, AIDS and well woman clinics – may not have been present then but the basis of the policy was not new. It appeared that all Michael Meacher's hard-working study groups and their detailed proposals had disappeared from the immediate agenda (and Meacher himself was to lose the health portfolio after the election).

The Alliance, with its ill-fated title of *Britain United. The Time Has Come* (Social Democratic Party, Liberal Alliance 1987) offered an increase in the NHS budget of £1 billion a year in five years, cuts in hospital waiting lists, more screening and well woman clinics and the banning of tobacco advertising. It wished to extend patients' rights. It planned to make care in the community a reality by providing extra funding, enlisting paid carers for the elderly and handicapped, and providing holidays for families caring for a member at home. The manifesto recognized a right to private medicine, but not the private use of NHS facilities at subsidized cost.

The Alliance policy intentions had been spelled out in more detail in a pamphlet (SDP 1987). This proposed an innovation fund with a budget of £250 million and offered the promise of funding for reforms in nurse education, in line with proposals identified in Project 2000, a plan to rationalize nurse training welcomed by the Royal College of Nursing (*Guardian*, 2 May 1988). The private sector would be charged a bed levy to help pay for the training and other assistance they derived from the NHS. Regional health authorities would be brought under elected regional authorities.

To return to the Labour Party, one of the best (and for Labour supporters one of the more distressing) analyses of Labour's defeat was published in April – before the date of the election was known and the campaign had begun! Raphael Samuel (*Guardian*, 20 April 1987) criticized Labour's failure to dent the government's arguments on public expenditure even in an area where it would have appeared vulnerable and in which there would have been much popular antagonism to cuts, an area such as the NHS. Further, Labour defended the public services as they existed and did not propose structural changes in the way they were run, even in those areas where they manifestly failed to meet changing needs. With regard to the NHS, we have seen that it was not an absence of ideas but a failure of these to be translated into clear policy commitments. For example, there appeared no policy initiatives in an area where so much material was becoming available – class inequalities in health and the failure of the NHS in its established form to dent these. 'Electorally speaking, Labour has chosen to travel light', according to Samuel.

Perhaps the avoidance of ideas concerning the organization of the NHS and the reformulation of what party policy should be fell victim of an overriding concern with a fear of being labelled extremist. Labour had enthusiastically accepted this Conservative-generated spectre. This meant that Labour, already on the defensive, had to enter the election by discarding its 'vote losing policies and establishing its bona fides'. The tendency (unfortunate choice of words!) was to play safe and it did this either by an appeal to a tired rhetoric or by an attack on the government that appeared to concentrate on a sterile dispute about the true figures, for example on health spending. Such a position would never allow an Opposition to seize the initiative.

Samuel described Labour's policy-makers as

a new race of political know alls who make a profession of their forensic skills – agnostics posing as realists, born again moderates building a whole politics out of nicely calculated less and more; British Gramscians practising tactics for all the world as if they were engaged in a war of position or manoeuvre rather than beating an abject retreat... Strategy these days is something approaching an obsession on the left, a surrogate for conviction.

As with many previous elections the opinion polls figured large in identifying issues and so shaping party presentation. One poll asked what the most important issue in the election was; 40 per cent of respondents answered 'health' (about the same proportion as answered 'unemployment'). Labour had a clear lead over the Conservatives in terms of public perception of their commitment to the NHS. A clear majority said they were prepared to see taxes increased and more money thus spent on the NHS when they were asked 'what is best for the country'. When asked 'what is best for you and your family' the proportion who favoured increased taxes for more NHS spending and those that did not were about equal (*The Politics of Choice*, BBC Radio 4, 26 May 1987).

The Conservatives maintained their stance of being the true supporters of the NHS and quoted many figures in the campaign. They kept the argument simple – we are spending more than has ever been spent. Some of their supporters from within the medical profession were keen to develop this simple message and argue, for example, that the problems evident in some acute areas were the result of the long-term commitment to shift funds to the care of the mentally ill, the mentally handicapped and the elderly, or to argue about the geographical redistribution of health resources. But generally government politicians did not venture into explanation or justification save for the ritual recitation of the 'figures'.

This stance led the Labour Party to decide that it had to challenge the Conservatives' claims. The result was a defensive posture that failed to present a coherent alternative strategy. Labour speakers would say that, although the Conservatives claim to be spending more, they are not in fact doing so – but Labour would spend more. Brian Gould, Labour's campaign manager, on BBC Radio 4's 'Election Call' (18 May 1987) provided an example of the difficulty such a stance creates. When asked to respond to the Conservatives' spending figures he made two points, both no doubt valid but neither really convincing as the grounds for an alternative policy. He suggested the reality of the NHS today could be ascertained by asking its staff. In addition, he said that the Conservatives' figures on the rate of increase in spending looked better than they were because they chose 1981 as a base. This ignored the considerable damage done to the NHS between 1979 and 1981. This sort of pedantic technocratism did not succeed in shifting the focus of debate, which surely Labour needed to do. The initiative remained with the Conservatives. One is reminded of criticisms of the Attlee government that they thought of socialism as a continuation of wartime central planning rather than as a mandate for social change (Channel 4 TV *The People's Flag*, 9 November 1987).

The Alliance, in its election broadcast on 18 May, adopted an interesting position. They stressed that the NHS should be understood as a moral enterprise (in contrast to something dominated by considerations of finance and debates about levels of funding). It was, David Owen argued, essentially about a perception of the many caring for the few.

Arguments about health charges and about privatization featured during the campaign. The opposition parties thought that they had a chance to exploit a Conservative vulnerability after Mrs Thatcher told a press conference that she chose private health care for herself because she wanted to exercise her right as a citizen to have treatment on the day and time she wanted and with the doctor of her choice. But once again such personalizing did not allow for any developed critique of the impact of privatization and private health on the nature of service offered by the NHS. It was not Mrs Thatcher's exercise of choice that was the key issue but what her choice does to other people who are not able to exercise that degree of control over their health care.

Underlying issues raised during the election campaign included arguments by the opposition that the crisis in the NHS was both of finance and of morale. Certainly there appeared to be a considerable degree of dissatisfaction among staff about conditions of service. For some this focused on pay. It had not just been about levels of pay but also about the continuing practice (although not in the election year) of holding back agreed pay deals. Also of considerable concern was the rhetoric of the government in linking pay increases above the inflation rate with money taken out of direct facilities for patients.

Some commentators saw the greatest problem for the NHS as being one of staffing. They pointed to the situation in central London where there were major problems in recruiting and keeping nurses and where 30 per cent of nurses were agency nurses. For others it was the introduction of the general manager and the cult of management in general. This, they argued, far from removing waste and maximizing efficiency, had led to a particularly narrow concern with performance – defined managerially not medically. Performance indicators, efficiency savings and performance-related bonuses had all taken the service too far, it was argued. Perhaps the first round of economies did identify some areas of waste – it would be a surprise if such a large organization did not have the capacity for improvement. But the repeat prescription, year after year, was now leading to a questioning of quality of care factors that were not quantifiable, but were deeply felt within the NHS: issues like having sufficient staff on a ward to allow nurses time to talk to both patients and to each other.

Other important impacts on morale included the rise of private medicine, creating a two-tier system within the professions who staffed the NHS. This included the presence of 'moonlighters' making considerable personal profit at a time when the larger staff community saw low pay and inadequate resources still prevalent in the NHS.

As to the funding debate, I have gone into this and tried to present the essence of the dispute on figures. That the centre of the argument had remained this rather than the observed and documented deterioration and continuing class differentials in health seemed to illustrate the agenda-setting power of the party in power. Even in discussing actual expenditure the government chose to emphasize its capital programme – Norman Fowler waving a long computerized list of hospital building projects was, as mentioned earlier, a high spot of the Conservative Party Conference. The real growth in capital spending was about 6.5 per cent per year over the previous six years and as such was considerably more than increases in revenue spending.

But even this figure was suspect. The House of Commons Social Services Committee (1986b) had criticized 'slippage' in the capital programme. This meant that projects might have been started, and so appear on lists like that of the Secretary of State, but they were either not finished or when finished stood empty because the revenue to operationalize them was not available. Seventeen major capital schemes due to start in 1986-7 included seven which were supposed to have started in 1985-6. Land sales were financing 15 per cent of the NHS capital programme (King's Fund 1987a).

One of the paradoxes of the relative generosity towards the capital programme was that the government's policy emphasis on care in the community, and the increasing demands for services for the elderly in particular, appeared best served by an expansion in revenue spending, in providing more staff for these labour-intensive activities.

On general spending, the weight of informed argument was increasingly that changing population structure (1 per cent), increased costs of new medicines and medical technology (0.5 per cent) and the development costs of meeting new government priorities such as more screening, more kidney and heart treatment, or longer-term commitments like the community care of the mentally ill (0.5 per cent) required together a real increase in spending of 2 per cent per year to maintain the quality of service offered. As always, at issue here was how far efficiency savings had closed the gap between what was provided and what was needed. The balance of opinion outside the DHSS appeared to be that just taking population changes and new technology into account produced a realization that real resources available to health authorities had been falling for much of the post-1979 period. Further, the effects of redistribution via RAWP were such as to make the situation in some districts severe. Even taking into account the 'gains' of competitive tendering and efficiency saving the levels of spending had not reached positive growth. Further, the indications were that the big savings had been made and any more would be essentially at the margin.

The number of people covered by private health insurance had doubled since 1979 to 5.2 million, nearly 10 per cent of the population. About £600 million was now spent annually on private health care. Much of this increase had been generated by companies insuring their employees. It did appear that the private sector was stimulated either by the perceived problems of the NHS or by real shortcomings. For example, a quarter of all hip replacement operations were carried out privately. In total about 15 per cent of non-emergency surgery was carried out in private hospitals and the pattern of demand for such surgery often reflected the length of waiting lists for similar surgery under the NHS. There were now 198 private acute hospitals in the United Kingdom with 10,000 beds, a 50 per cent increase since 1979. Some spare capacity was evident, particularly in London. It was evident that, for serious complaints, 40 per cent of people with private health insurance still went to the NHS. But the general trend throughout the country was for an expansion of private facilities. The private sector had also breached the walls of the NHS in areas other than the 3000 pay beds still in existence. For example, BUPA bought a machine for treating and getting rid of kidney stones without surgery, located in St Thomas's Hospital, London. Treatment cost £2000 per patient in the private sector and the waiting list in the NHS was between two and three years.

I have looked in detail at arguments around the provision of private medicine. To conclude, we can note the pleas from some private companies that to expand they needed the help of the government, particularly in granting tax advantages for private health insurance premiums. This can be compared with an interesting plea for government intervention to promote the 'free market' by one NHS worker interviewed on radio (*File on Four*, BBC Radio 4, 28 October 1987). He suggested that if the government wanted competition it should not tie the hands of the NHS. One central London teaching hospital could be converted into NHS PLC and staffed by NHS consultants who, as part of their contract with the NHS, would agree to work in this part of the private sector. It would then compete with the rest of the private sector and according to him 'wipe it out almost immediately'. Funds raised by NHS PLC could then by recycled in the NHS!

PART III

Putting the Policy into Practice

8 Planning in the National Health Service

Having examined the politics of health policy-making as it is evident in the formal decision-making structures and as it is presented in the public debate of the media I now move on to examine features of the way that policy is put into practice. I will look, in particular, at planning and management as presenting two spheres of activity and at economics and business as approved of constructs.

Planning in the NHS is difficult to define. Perhaps we can best understand planning as being what planners do. What planners say they do not do is either make policy or manage its implementation. Planners act in accordance with planning theory, or planning theory accords with what planners do. Such solipsisms serve only to keep us some distance from the experienced reality of planning. What we can say is that social practice on the part of planners helps set the parameters of debate about the feasibility of particular options in the policy-making process. But policy-making and the administration of policy-making transcend the confines of planners and planning theory. Perhaps the key question to ask, therefore, is the extent to which, in the NHS, the planning process is proactive or reactive. It appears almost axiomatic that planning to be planning must be future-orientated (Hearn 1982, p. 161) but this is an assumption we must test against the detail of observed practice.

The implication of an understanding of planning as an activity relating to self-conscious activity and self-definition is that we must examine it as we would examine an ideological construct. Further, if we understand planning as ideology then how far does this determine its agenda-setting function? Given these general observations it is appropriate to study practice and the beliefs and meanings attributed to that practice.

Kemp (1982) identified current orthodoxies in planning theory and practice as primarily adopting a mode of rationality that emphasizes the instrumental and the technical. This underlines a positivism that is concerned with control and the maintenance of the status quo. There is a preoccupation with the need to predict from existing states of affairs and a reluctance either to question fundamental assumptions or to examine the aspects of planning that might emphasize responsiveness or accountability as opposed to performance. It is not that planners develop this sort of practice by themselves. They are influenced by the prevailing paradigms of the time.

Planning is often seen as a mechanism used by the state as a device to further its legitimation needs. This may be characterized by a process of depoliticizing the planning arena. Perhaps a process of consultation will be used that essentially serves the function of incorporating other groups and other views as opposed to developing a responsiveness to them. Further, it may be that the very language used includes distortions and repressions and so planning as a communicative process may have been distorted by political ideology and may run the risk of neither being comprehensible nor sincere (Habermas 1979).

Other critiques are wary of abstracting planning as an entity choosing to emphasise the importance of understanding totalities. Alain Touraine (1974) argues that

> Whether the economy is conceived in terms of planning or a firm is seen as a decision-making system, strict sociological analysis demonstrates the increasing dependence of the conditions of development on the entire structure of social organisation.

He argues that social life cannot be understood by an analysis of function and to seek an understanding of social behaviour as something governed by norms and values translated into institutions attributes a permanence to what is essentially transitory. What is central is to look at the mechanisms of influence and of negotiation, the way individuals and collectivities seek solutions and pursue objectives.

In developing these arguments, he is addressing the same problematic as Ralf Dahrendorf, whose project appears to be to evolve a theory of conflict in industrial society that takes cognizance of the dynamic theories of nineteenth-century sociology, particularly that of Marx. These primarily related men's behaviour to their economic position. To these he wished to add twentieth-century sociology's concern with how social groups cohere. Like Habermas and like Touraine, although with a different set of assumptions and understandings, he speaks of the importance of studying forces operating from within and without organizational structures; he calls them exogenous and endogenous structures (Dahrendorf 1959, p. 127). For him social conflict is far from a random occurrence, it is rather an outgrowth of the structure of a given society.

There will exist latent and manifest interests within what Max Weber called 'imperatively co-ordinated associations' (quoted in Dahrendorf 1959, p. 167). These may, in many cases, be identified as an antagonistic interaction between dominant and subordinate layers in the authority structure (Roy 1968).

Touraine is concerned to identify the nature of conflict and he is critical of reductionist arguments that, for example, reduce conflict to economics. Many economic decisions, he says, are made not out of consideration of profit but on the basis of expansion and power. Of course, the dilemma here is one of the time-scale used. We might argue that economic reward can be deferred and short-term gains set against long-term possibilities.

Much of his work has been designed to discuss the nature of oppositional movements and here he also makes contributions of considerable value for a study of the NHS. He identifies a phenomenon of dependent participation whereby alienation cancels out social conflict. This is encouraged and supported by the prevailing structure of social domination pressurizing the individual into participating, controlling needs and attitudes and taking the initiative via an agenda-setting political aggressiveness. The likelihood in such situations is that oppositional movements will lag behind the speed of social change and base their programmes on analyses dating from earlier situations. They will insist on a continuity between the great battles of the past and those of the present. He contrasts this with social movements like Poland's Solidarity whose most vital function is to present a model of democratic practice and in so doing to pose an alternative to the bureaucratic state (Touraine 1983). It is that one has to transcend the parameters of the possible, as defined by the state, in order effectively to challenge it on any but the most superficial issues.

As well as identifying the shortcomings of many social movements, he is critical of sociology that, like them, has lagged behind the dynamic of social change. It may have been appropriate to study the social and political regulation of capitalism in the early days and certainly Durkheim's attempts to study the nature of social solidarity appeared crucial for sociology at that time. But to retain a sociology that is separate from the action of economic transformation and that remains concerned with norms and values, and to assume these are manifest in institutional structure, is to miss the possibilities of studying mechanisms of influence and negotation. In so doing one loses the opportunity to be interested in objectives as opposed to second-order phenomena like values.

Getting nearer to planning as action and as theory, we can see the problems inherent in defining planning as being anything other than a means for serving the dominant paradigms and the interests of what is, rather than what could be. This is not a surprising observation and one might ask why planning is being asked to do anything more. Surely the focus of the structure in dominance is elsewhere. A study of power should be geared towards the political and economic structure of the state, or towards the totality in action.

But the impact of planning is important in giving legitimacy to the situation as it is and in helping define the parameters of the possible, not just for the dominant power structure but also for oppositional movements. When a particular definition of reality, of the possible, is attached to a concrete power it is called ideology (Berger and Luckman 1966). Such ideologies are, in effect, historical structures and cultural objects rather than just states of consciousness. Althusser (1977, p. 233) argues that 'Men "live" their ideologies as the Cartesians "saw" . . . the moon two hundred paces away, not at all as a form of consciousness but as an object of their world'. They are analysable, therefore, independently of their material origin.

Specific examples of ways of conceptualizing planning which illustrate the importance of ideology might include a distinction between conservative ideologies, which reduce problems to particulars, and radical ideologies, which generalize symptoms into wider problems – thus always demanding more action (Bailey 1975, p. 33). For the former the problems of a deteriorating class differential in general health might be responded to by offering the evidence of increased spending on, say, hospital building or screening. The latter might deny that progress in such areas was centrally relevant but still say that all that can be done is to have more resources, without a critique of why increases in resources in the past have not produced the results desired.

Extending such approaches to the establishment of the NHS, we could argue that this was seen as not so much an opportunity for change in society as a justified expansion of the state into public life. That it did also produce change, of sorts, was a second-order result. The NHS served the role of justifying a certain form of social organization and social knowledge. It has not challenged dominant paradigms.

We might compare it with the experience of health care in other countries. For example, the development of the rural health workers' service in Tanzania was done in such a way as to emphasize independent practice and autonomy rather than the alternative model which would have seen them as yet another arm of the state intruding into the lives of the previously private world of the people (Skeet 1978, pp. 110–20; see also Werner 1978, for a powerful comparison of the ideal primary health worker and the conventional doctor). Or the decision of the Nicaraguan government to refuse a hospital funded by the World Health Organization because it would have led to the development of a technocratic, urban-based, medical service that would not have empowered the people (Escudero 1980). Technocratic medicine may have benefited some people but to embrace it means embracing far more. The danger lies in establishing a model of relationships between the experts, the professions and the government that is hierarchic and exclusive. These dangers outweigh the benefits.

Such a perception of health, and the opportunities it presents for health planning, have been largely absent in the United Kingdom. This is in part explained by a first world myopia which denies even the possibility of learning from outside the Europe/North America axis. The exception is evident in some approaches from community health groups (for example, the work of the Community Health Initiatives Resource Unit, 26 Bedford Square, London WC1), neighbourhood groups (for example, the work in Brent publicized by its Community Health Council including 'The Struggle for Brent's Health Service', 'It's my life doctor', and 'This is what we want'; Brent CHC can be contacted at 16 High Street, London NW10), ethnic groups ('Black People and the Health Service', again from Brent) and the women's health movement (see Rodmell and Watt 1986). In some cases these have identified the structure and dominant practice of health care as being an intrinsic part of their problem – to be combated as ill health is combated.

Other examples of radical practice include responses to mental illness from anti-psychiatry (Boyers and Orrill 1972), patients' self-help (Mental Patients Union; see also MIND, 22 Harley Street, London W1) and therapeutic communities (Hinshelwood and Manning 1979). But nowhere in the United Kingdom has there been the sort of sustained critique of practice vis-à-vis the mentally ill as there has been in Italy. There the institutional politics of mental health was firmly associated with dominant power structures in the rest of society. Franco Basaglia's (1981) criticisms of practice centred on an analysis that said the very existence of the asylum establishes a dynamic of oppression between the doctor and the patient. The asylum cannot be transformed, it has to be abolished. This is a very much more sophisticated analysis than the meandering debates over British community care (see Lovell 1978).

The lack of a radical critique of health and of the NHS in the United Kingdom may, in part, be attributed to the continuing ambivalence about examining what has been ideologically constructed as the 'jewel in Labour's crown', or as an example of socialism in practice. It is as if the belief on the Left is that the NHS is sufficiently under attack from the Right and in such an environment its friends keep quiet about their own doubts. I have argued that this serves only to place the Left on the defensive and that a sustained analysis of the NHS and its shortcomings might strengthen its support (albeit via reconstructing a more appropriate service).

If the NHS serves as an icon for the Labour Party and as a comforting ideological construct for many in the population it is its workers who perhaps identify its shortcomings most readily. To many of them the establishment of a National Health Service, just like the process of nationalization, was designed to let things continue as they were. It was to support the status quo and certainly not to present a model of social change or of a different relationship between employer and staff. The result, in many cases, has been to stifle interest in public ownership because it becomes identified with outmoded and restrictive practice and with labour relations like those of the private sector. The story of a prevalent sense of betrayal when miners discovered that the pit bosses of the new National Coal Board were, in many cases, the same people as the old bosses of the private coal companies is a story perhaps distorted and embellished in its repeated telling – but none the less true. In the NHS, from very early on, the staff and in particular the nurses had a perception of a service in crisis and a service built on the exploited labour of such as themselves – trapped by a public myth of their role as much as by low pay and tied accommodation (Menzies 1960; Baly 1987).

If the NHS is locked into a dominant paradigm of planning and what is is mistaken for what must be, give or take a few million pounds, we still can study it both for itself and as a manifestation of a particular ideology. It is not an easy organizational structure to study for the policy-making system's main characteristics, according to David Hunter (1980), are centralization, exclusiveness, secrecy, corporatism, authoritarianism, and an emphasis on administrative primacy. Even these might not be bad enough but we also must ask if this elaborate edifice of policy-making is a sham. Perhaps 'The cynical view is...realistic; reform arises from political demands or political expediency, and the language of rational discovery is a façade' (Stanyer and Smith 1976, p. 266).

So as not to stop in disarray I will remind myself of the early history of planning which is described by Bailey (1975, p. 35) as evidencing a 'bifurcation of reform into utopianist comprehensiveness (Owen, Salt, Howard, etc.) on the one hand and the technical remedialism of the late nineteenth century on the other'. Public health reforms were adopted in a largely piecemeal fashion, dependent upon the enthusiasm of the relevant local authority for their implementation. Central government was reluctant to intervene to set national standards or to plan services over wide areas. Much of the initiative came from experts and much of the appeal of reform was related to a technocratic wish to 'conquer nature' coupled with a wish for a healthy and profit-generating workforce and an underlying fear of the mob.

Public health aside, the rest of health care emerged in a largely unplanned way, in the sense of more than one facility at a time being considered, until in the 1930s the Sankey Commission proposed the imposition of a centralized co-ordinating structure on public and voluntary hospital provision. The Commission went over much of the ground later to be incorporated in thinking on the establishment of the NHS – not that it envisaged this happening.

It appeared in the 1930s, in the United Kingdom as well as in other industrialized communities, that the depression brought about an inevitable increase in government intervention in the life of the people. In the United States the Tennessee Valley Authority and the New Deal fundamentally redefined this relationship. But developments in public works and in intervention in the economy and in industry did not lead to a planning strategy for the provision of health care. It was the onset of war in 1939 and the establishment of the Emergency Medical Service that did this.

The direction of labour and the central control of resources acted as a spur to the innovations that became codified in the National Health Service Act. After the war planning in the NHS was dominated by a quickly recognized shortage of funds for development, by the inherited problems of hospital stock in need of repair and modernization and by a geographical distribution that did not respond to the need then apparent. A history of planning in the NHS therefore would emphasize its being essentially remedial and reactive to changes in the broader political and economic world. It was also largely incremental.

Hospital provision was so expensive that it dominated discussion on health planning. Within the hospital sector the emphasis in development plans was placed on targets for achieving a certain number of acute hospital beds per 1000 of the population. Planners and administrators concentrated on this. At the same time medical orthodoxies were changing faster than hospital services could be provided. One result was that the 'ideal' size for hospitals went up and down, thus causing considerable disruption in 'Hospital Plans'.

If such planning was essentially reactive it was also experiencing problems in addressing areas which either transcended the boundaries of two or more ministries or included the spheres of competence of central and local government. An example was the absence of co-ordination between housing and health despite their location, for a time, within the same ministry.

Planning occurs within a particular 'action space' (Parston 1980, p. 79) and that space has been defined narrowly. It has, for example, excluded considerations of occupational health and in so doing has made any comprehensive service impossible. The realization that, in some cases, it is work that makes you sick has eluded health planners. When such issues have been addressed they have been presented as having specific aetiologies, and links with social structure and differential power have not been pursued. Cancer provides many appropriate examples. Where you work can greatly affect your chances of getting cancer. 'Workers in petrochemical, asbestos, steel smelting and some mining industries are particularly high risk groups' (Doyal 1983a, p. 132). Sometimes the connections are complex. One appears to be between industrial pollutants and cancer of the cervix. But the connection may be through the occupational status of the victim's husband. The typical victim of this cancer is 'an elderly woman who lived much of her life in a house without a bathroom and was married to a man who came home in dirty overalls' (Jean Robinson, quoted in Davey 1988, p. 33). Prolonged contact with oils, greases and metal dust associated with engines and machine tools and the general cleanliness of an occupation may be factors. Such speculative findings appear in reports on occupational mortality from the Office of Population Censuses and Surveys. But it is not just the complexity, and controversy, about the relative impact of these factors alongside others – sexual behaviour and smoking being two – but also the lack of any contact between such findings and the policy and planning apparatus of the NHS. Such findings do not intrude on its action space.

The dominance of the hospital sector is evident in the annual reports of the NHS in its early years. In 1952, for example, the revised estimate for the year 1951–2 of total expenditure on the NHS was £399,183,000; of this £213,483,013 was to be spent on hospital running costs, and £11,123,269 on hospital capital expenditure (Ministry of Health 1952). The capital expenditure figures are not indicative of spending on new plant but on the servicing needs of the old. No new hospitals were built to replace out-of-date ones or to serve the developing communities and new housing estates.

In the early years there was also a concern that the increase in demand was faster than that in resources allocated. One response was to plan for a more intense use of beds and encourage shorter stays in hospital. Policies from these early years, of course, have a resonance today. Between 1949 and 1956 the number of beds available increased by 6 per cent whereas the number of patients treated in them went up by 27 per cent. Staffing numbers did not keep pace (Ministry of Health 1957). The Ministry might offer the rationale of improved efficiency, or of the benefits to patients and their families of shorter periods in hospital, but with such a strong cost rationale one suspects that quality of service was not the dominant consideration.

The NHS, from its beginnings in hopeful adhocery, moved towards a model of planning which claimed the justification of rationality. But it had the central dilemma of trying to plan around, and with, the tripartite division of the service. The Guillebaud (1956) Committee and the Porritt Report (Medical Services Review Committee 1962) both addressed the weaknesses of such a system. The advantages of a single administrative structure, according to the Medical Services Review Committee (1962, para. 609), were that this would help 'produce regional and central operational research on which future planning and development of a service [could] be rationally based'. But a system as divided as this one reflected other imperatives, notably power, influence and the political struggle between government and the professions. To analyse it using only a construct of rationality is to ignore the reasons for its existence and the pattern of its development.

One dilemma in discussing the development of planning is that much of the debate has been predicated upon a dominant assumption that the task centres on how to spend increasing resources. But the reality has been rather that the NHS has had, in recent years, to spend time looking at how to prioritize existing services and evaluate demands for new ones in the light of either stationary or decreasing real resources and definitely reducing resources relative to need. One commentator (Eversley 1975, p. 26) suggests that 'Planning in an age of stagnation is not the mirror image of planning in an age of increase. It is an activity different in kind rather than in degree'. Hearn and Roberts (1975) agree and contrast what they call crisis management with rational planning. It is interesting to compare their description of a crisis scenario, and the decremental planning it creates, with the assumption – by inference – of what is the 'normal' process of planning. I would suggest that in the following quotation one could substitute normal for decremental and in so doing still present a convincing argument:

> Decremental planning is contentious, complex and time consuming, so it is likely that only a limited number of alternatives will be considered and that decision makers will tend to adopt the first one that appears good enough.

Hearn (1982, pp. 167–8) argues elsewhere that 'affluence may have fostered planning, but crisis has brought the plans themselves home to roost'. The danger in positing decrementalism as a different sort of activity is that this will, in contrast, give a structure and rationality to normal planning that it does not possess.

Essentially decrementalism (the process of directly or indirectly planning for small reductions or decrements, as opposed to incrementalism, which affects small increments) 'results from the interplay of technocratic responses to the bourgeois pressure to limit and restructure the state' (Hearn 1982, p. 168). Hearn identifies five major forms of decrementalism. The first is *planning abandoned*, where there is an emphasis on fast decisions made by a few. The decisions are directly linked with the outcomes to be achieved, for example a reduction in the number of staff, and not related to the identifiable purpose of the organization. This form is usually accompanied by the discovery of crisis which is used to justify the action and the mechanism by which the action was taken. The creation of a language of crisis makes this process easier. In recent years this language has been promoted by the critics of the government who in so heightening the debate make arbitrary action by the government both easier and more likely to be accepted. The second form of decrementalism is *expedient planning*, where crisis is assumed to be imminent rather than present and where consequently planning concentrates on attempting what is considered most likely to be accepted and achieved as opposed to what is most needed. The third is *crisis planning*, which is not as reactive as planning abandoned and expedient planning and purports to a proactive and rationalist stance. But crisis planning which anticipates future demands on a service may occur alongside cuts in other key related services. For example, health authorities may plan for the likely future costs of treating people with AIDS but at the same time reduce expenditure on support for patients in the community. Who defines what is a crisis and so deserves this sort of contingency planning is of key importance. The fourth form of decremantalism is *strategic planning*, where the realization of potential crisis requires an informed rethinking of both the planning process and the dominant planning objectives. Within this type the political and ideological process of setting new objectives is crucial, although it may be presented as a manifestation of rationality. The fifth type is *persistent planning*, which is a powerful pressure to carry on regardless, not to acknowledge crisis, 'to plough ahead with "doing" planning as in more settled times, but to ignore its implications and prescriptions, to say one thing and do another', to believe usual practice can be observed and then to express surprise when aspired for plans do not materialize. It is of great importance to consider such an activity in any investigation of strategic planning in the NHS. Bosanquet (1980) described the response of the NHS to an atmosphere of cash control and cutback:

> Locally the NHS is still acting as if this was all an unfortunate intermission. Planning teams go on pumping out plans for large capital schemes and increases in staff. It is still assumed that increases in services for the elderly, the mentally ill and the mentally handicapped can be financed out of a growth element which has all but disappeared . . . On the 'business as usual' approach, the NHS would come to provide an increasingly inappropriate service in ageing buildings. Planning would serve as a release through fantasy.

At this point it does seem important to look at some dimensions of the NHS that impinge upon its providing a straightforward analysis of either incrementalism or decrementalism. The first is to remind ourselves that incrementalism developed as a means of understanding the budgetary process and perhaps we would want to distinguish between budgeting and planning. The second is that we must impose a time structure on what we identify as planning. The NHS now operates with two sorts of plan – strategic and operational. Formally, the latter ought to be concerned with the detailed implementation of the former. But in practice they appear to be based on two different, but related, sets of financial assumptions.

According to incremental theory a budget consists largely of a repetition of the budget which preceded it the year before. Budgeting consists of adding a marginal increment (decrement). It is therefore not about a comprehensive review of bids from different parts of the organization. Nor is it about rational decision-making matching resources to identified need (Dahl and Lindblom 1953). The plausibility of the theory, Wildavsky (1964) asserts, is evident from an appreciation that, given the complexity of issues at stake, decision-makers have only very limited time. They have limited knowledge and intellectual capacity to do anything more than consider procedures such as standardized but marginal increases, or decreases, to last year's allocation.

But budgeting and planning in the NHS go on in an environment where the dominance of political debate is such as to set agendas not apparently amenable to straightforward incrementalism or decrementalism. For example, it may be that something that has entered the public realm as a subject of popular disquiet will receive funds and these may be allocated at the expense of incremental planning. The government's political decision to reduce waiting lists and to concentrate on certain areas of need it felt most likely to produce quick changes in numbers is a case in point. It did not link with long-term strategic plans, or with the disposition of capital resources by health authorities. It required an adjustment of already determined priorities.

There is evident a real split in understanding between economists developing models of decision-making, policy analysts and planners. One writer who has attempted to bridge the gap is P.M. Jackson (1982). He makes the perceptive point that interdisciplinary co-operation, or indeed thinking, is inhibited by a reluctance to stray outside the security of an often hard-gained expertise.

The Nobel Prize winning economist, Herbert Simon, criticizes the assumption of a pursuit of a 'rational maximizing solution' by saying that the machinery for seeking that solution is not available. He suggests that planners do not have enough time to look for the sharpest needle in the haystack but for the first they come across one that is just sharp enough. They are faced with the dilemma of how to include in calculations that purport to rationality, factors such as social cost as well as economic cost, how to measure efficiency in such a way as to include demand-side as well as supply-side calculations, how to include quality as a factor in assessing efficiency and performance, and how to develop a model for a system where the marginal cost and the total cost exist in a very complex relationship because of the commitments to maintain fixed capital. On a purely cost-benefit analysis one may wish to close down old facilities that need a great deal of money to be spent simply in upkeep, but find that such facilities cannot be closed because there are no comparable units offering the same sort of care within a particular geographical area and because costing does not allow for a new facility to be built.

Planners have responded to the identification of such difficulties in reconciling complexities. They have considered ways to measure efficiency and ways to create equations that allow different demands to be balanced. But in general it is still fair to say that the economics of planning operates with the heuristic fiction that the task relates to a utility-maximizing individual who faces only budgetary constraints. There is not a recognition of uncertainty in the environment nor of problems with obtaining adequate and even-handed information.

But this is only one of many heuristic fictions evident in planning – at times the process appears to be of the sort that would be safer if everyone spoke a different language so that there would be less fear of misbelieving that we understand what they are saying (to borrow an observation made in writing about what goes on in group meetings by Bion 1968).

The splits between cultures operating within the same organizational framework used to be identified as those between the sciences and the humanities but now may be centred on different distinctions. Bennis (1970) offered an alternative:

> Like C.P. Snow, I feel that there is a growing separation of the two isolated cultures. However, I speak not of the chasm between scientist and humanist, but of that between men with knowledge who lack power and men with power who lack knowledge.

In health planning this is further complicated by doubts about what is the most important form of knowledge and about a distinction between different sorts of power. For example, is it more important to know about the constraints of financial exigencies and what can realistically be aspired to. Or is it more important to know what can be done – and needs to be provided to ensure its being done successfully – in terms of medical technique? In considering power there is an important distinction between initiatory capacity and negative power, the power to prevent change through non-cooperation. In all discussions about social policy, and certainly in the NHS, it is important to consider negative power and the importance of non-decisions. What is not included in the decision-making process and what is not presented because of a belief that it would never get through, as well as what appears to have been decided but then never materializes, are as important to understand as what does appear in planning documents and what is popularly agreed to represent objectives.

A further complication to the incrementalism/decrementalism model, as it relates to health, lies in this need to assess the central role played by the medical profession. Hence we have to include in any analysis an assessment of its influence. Ideologically and organizationally the medical profession have been centrally located in the establishment and subsequent evolution of the NHS. A key factor underlying this central role has been the notion of 'clinical freedom'. In seeking to understand planning it is an important phenomenon to examine because it appears to exist outside the normal planning paradigms. It certainly exists beyond a narrow economist's definition of utility and cost, and hence rationality.

There have been attempts to incorporate clinicians' perceptions into an overall planning agenda. But these attempts have depended upon the success of convincing doctors to give up some part of what they traditionally considered as within the scope of clinical freedom. There have been not only attempts to introduce some measure of economic 'logic' in the form of clinical budgeting and QALYs but also numerous exhortations to doctors that they should seek to understand management and its problems and possibilities. I will consider all the features of the debate but, first, will comment on the variety of medical practice that results from the exercise of clinical freedom.

Michael Cooper (1975) has provided a summary of some of the issues raised; for example, he points to the problems created when general practice and hospital services are not planned together. This is, in part, a problem inherent in the tripartite division of the NHS but is also linked with clinical and organizational freedom for doctors. He cites an example where one general practice introduced an appointment system; the impact of this was seen not just in the surgery but in the local hospital's accident and emergency department, where attendance from the area covered by the practice in question increased by 50 per cent. More generally, it is a commonplace that approximately 70 per cent of the workload of casualty departments could be adequately dealt with by GPs.

The relationship between GPs and hospital specialists varies greatly. One study in Edinburgh found the rate of referral from general practice to specialist to vary between 0.6 per cent and 25.8 per cent of patients.

Once in hospital both the kinds of treatment and its length can vary considerably. Even after applying standardization for age and sex the length of stay following appendicitis varies by a factor of six. (A 1971 study of West German medical practice discovered an appendectomy performance rate three times higher than that for any other country; at the same time another study found that of these only one in four patients given the operation had indeed been suffering from appendicitis! (Lichtner and Pflanz 1971)) Staying with some international comparisons, in the United States a planning technique involves developing patterns of treatment that will ensure an average hospital stay that permits each bed to be used by 27 cases per year. If such a system were introduced in France it would be able to manage its workload with only 55 per cent of current hospital capacity.

The evidence from the United Kingdom would suggest that those consultants who insist on using more resources for their patients are not materially improving their condition. The treatment of hernias provides an example. Discharge after one day seemed to have no observable deleterious effect on patients as compared with discharge after a week. But at the time of this particular research, 1968, the average stay for this condition was 11 days, with some hospital groups averaging 21 (Cooper 1975).

The documentation identifying variations in diagnosis and in treatment is now considerable. There is also much literature on the prevalence of iatrogenic disease, that which results from the activity of physicians. It is Ivan Illich (1977) who has brought much of this body of data together. One example is the work of Solomon who cured confused and forgetful over-50s by denying them their usual prescribed doses of barbiturates (Cooper 1975, p. 57).

There are undoubtedly problems both in achieving a sufficient degree of systematic research on the efficacy of particular medical techniques and in disseminating such findings as there are. Some of these problems arise from both methodological and ethical reservations about, for example, the use of control groups (although some issues like the efficacy of bed rest would seem particularly amenable to control group research and would have considerable relevance in terms of the use of NHS resources).

It is a debate that varies with time; for example, the medical profession and the pharmaceutical industry have been criticized for allowing products to come onto the market before their long-term effects have been properly assessed. Thalidomide in the United Kingdom and Stilbestrol in the United States are only two of many examples. But they have been criticized recently for a preoccupation with playing safe in such a way as to withhold treatment from patients for whom no other treatment is available save a new, not yet fully tested, drug. This has occurred as one of the effects of the desperation felt by some people with AIDS. They argue that the choice about treatment ought to be their own. They may be prepared to accept a particular treatment because the length of time for proper testing is longer than the life expectancy of most of them. Clearly there is a complex issue in the nature of informed choice, civil liberties, the protection of the public and the correct haste for products to be made available to those in real need. What is debatable is whether the fear of litigation has meant that the process now takes too long.

The medical profession is certainly subject to considerable anxiety about the threat of the law and will change its practice in the face of the law's interventions. In the United States, for example, the proportion of babies born by Caesarian section is very high, and is rising. This would seem to be directly linked to a fear of litigation should damage be evident to a baby born normally. Caesarians are preemptive strikes to allay the possibility that doctors will be accused of not intervening enough and hence being deemed negligent. In the United Kingdom the dispute concerning the suspension of Wendy Savage, as well as being about a struggle over who controls childbirth – mothers or doctors – and whether childbirth was essentially a vital area for the imposition of the panoply of medical technology or whether medicine should be an occasional adjunct to an otherwise normal process, was about the perceived need to be seen to be doing something to allay the possibilities of litigation (Savage 1986).

Fundamentally the problem lies in a combination of the ideology of medicine and its structural position. The doctor is both the definer of need and the arbiter of treatment. As well as being designed to ensure the independence of medicine from the encroachment of other groups and to enshrine the perception of the medical profession as being synonymous with the pursuit of health and the appropriate treatment of illness, clinical freedom ensures a great variation in the interpretation of need, great inconsistences in treatment and an allocation, without challenge, of scarce resources to medical practice of no, or of disputed, value. Cooper (1975, p. 59) poses health planners three questions. First, can any benefit for the patient be identified in the existence and exercise of clinical freedom? Second, what level of resources can the state afford to allocate to eccentricities that result? Third, is such 'heroic individualism inconsistent with modern management'?

Before considering recent attempts to incorporate doctors' decision-making capability into a wider management framework, I will look at some other possible influences on planners that one might imagine would counterbalance the medical. Throughout the history of the NHS there have existed wider indicators of health and illness drawn up by epidemiologists. Prior to the Second World War they concentrated their attentions on the infectious diseases, in particular on identifying the characteristics distinguishing those suffering from particular conditions and the specific respects in which they differed *vis-à-vis* the general population. They offered a direct link between statistical observation and medical practice in an area where medical intervention seemed to have rapid results (Florey and Weddell 1976, p. 19). A more detailed reading of the history of infectious diseases and the social response to them underlines the importance of both environment and behavioural change.

But it remains the case that the rapid defeat of many widespread and deadly conditions supported a dominant construction of the potential omnipotence of medicine and of the value of teamwork between the epidemiologist and the clinician. It is perhaps salutory to remind ourselves that such an alliance had its recommendations transmitted into policy not just because of the appeal of science and of demonstrable achievement but also because of the lack of social discrimination by the infectious diseases. It was the socially promiscuous cholera germ that first galvanized Parliament into public health legislation.

The general decline in the prevalence of infectious diseases after the Second World War left a lot of underemployed epidemiologists. In so doing it allowed them the possibility of engaging in both a study of chronic disease and an investigation of patterns of disease as they related to specific population groups. These studies placed the epidemiologists, previously much approved of, in a position of likely conflict with politicians, policy-makers, planners and, potentially, doctors. The dilemma, as compared with infectious diseases, was that the conditions now being studied were not single-cause complaints and the recommendations about responses to them embraced the social as well as the medical. Or the recommendations might involve a much longer-term planning need where the results of spending input would not be readily apparent for a considerable time. For example, in the first case they might study links between unemployment and ill-health, and in the second they might underline the efficacy of mass screening for a number of conditions. Both recommendations would place them in the realm of dispute over social planning and public expenditure.

An indication of the impact of such a change in the fortunes of the hap-less epidemiologist is the extent to which his or her work is now either the centre of controversy or is subject to widespread criticism of its veracity and/or usefulness. We have seen in our review of the public expressions of health policy the number of times that reports have not been published, have not been disseminated widely by the sponsoring body, or have excited widespread critical (if not always well-informed) comment. The Black Report (Townsend and Davidson 1982), and the response it generated, remains the most apposite case. One thing this changed climate has generated is a sort of epidemiological 'counter culture' out to disprove the direct tie in between class and morbidity and mortality.

The development and spread of computing in the 1960s coincided with the popularization of the 'white heat of the technological revolution' as a political slogan. It appeared that politicians hoped an increasingly com-plex public sector decision-making process could be better informed by an improved flow of cogent social information. For example, social indicators, such as those of morbidity and mortality, could inform a programme designed to redistribute resource to areas in most need (that became the Resource Allocation Working Party, of which more shortly).

But the problems encountered in the use of this sort of social indicator were of two sorts. First, an apparent enthusiasm for better data did not hide the reality of a decision-making process that was still based on politics and not on the easy transmission of knowledge into action. There is a long and complex history of attempts to understand the links between knowledge and power. In Edward Said's brilliant book *Orientalism* (Said 1978; see also Said 1986) he analyses the affiliation of knowledge with power in discussing how the scholars of the period of empire helped to create an image of the East which provided the justification for the supremacist ideology of imperialism. The process of defining knowledge as being that which serves the establishment is also evident in the relationship of government to people within the United Kingdom. Knowledge is not knowledge if it does not serve the interests of the powerful, it is agitation or subversion. Policy-makers know what they wish to hear and they are very pleased to hear it. It allows them to present a different *raison d'être* for action, other than the pursuit of political objectives.

If the knowledge being made available is not consistent with these more over-riding needs it will be over-ridden. Looking at the issue of the evaluation of social care, Smith and Cantley (1985) point to problems that have arisen. If attempts at evaluation have made incorrect assumptions about the rational character of the policy process or about the nature of consensus in professional organizations, then they have directed their attention away from a proper consideration of the plurality of motive and of perspective which participants hold on service provision. Such is the case in relation also to privatization. I have described, in some detail, the situation in Cornwall where the health authority assumed that the dominant consideration was cost but discovered this to be subsumed by a wish to reduce the size of the workforce even if, in so doing, costs went up (see page 89).

The second main problem in the usefulness of social indicators is a methodological one. They all emphasize illness rather than health. When they move beyond a simple measurement of mortality they include an unmeasurable concept of good health which they translate into the measurable, but inadequate, surrogate of life expectancy. They then implicitly or explicitly postulate some theory of social behaviour which serves to relate the variables under consideration and to establish a correlation between concept and surrogate (Carley 1981, p. 174).

In addition to this level of methodological problem, there is a further one of the relationship between social pattern and individual choice. I have borrowed from Edward Said, writing in a different context, above and here will borrow from Alan Carling (1986, p. 27), also pursuing a rather different project but making, I think, some very useful observations for my analysis when he says:

> It has often seemed that there is one box marked agentless structure in which one peers to find modes of production, grand historical designs, epochal social change, ideological hegemony, sociological analysis, determinism and constraint, while one looks to another, marked 'structureless agency', to find the individual, volition and choice, moral judgement, politics-as-it-is-lived and history-as-it-is-experienced.

There have been two fruitful routes out of the impasse of these methodological shortcomings. The first is a move towards small-scale studies of health care provision in a particular city. This has allowed for a detailed study of the distribution of ill-health to be linked with the nature of the environment, the kinds of housing an area has, the distribution of industry, the pattern of local unemployment, and so on. These findings can then be linked with a study of the politics of the area and the priorities it has given to planning for health. Such multi-factoral, while detailed, studies of health seem to provide the closest approximation to understanding the way health facilities and health planning have both evolved and currently operate (see, for example, West of Scotland Politics of Health Group 1984, on Glasgow; and People's Campaign for Health 1984, on Sheffield). The other route, while not strictly concerned with epidemiology, seeks to evaluate according to the accounts of the legitimate subjects. Here the women's health movement has led the way (see Oakley and Graham 1982, Doyal 1983b, Boston Women's Health Book Collective 1984).

On a number of occasions in contemporary debate on the NHS the absence of annual reports of chief medical officers has been noted with regret. It is interesting to review the contents of these Reports and I will look at that from 1951 as an example of the contribution they did make, and might have continued to make, to the debate on health and ill-health (Ministry of Health 1951). The chief medical officer reviewed the general trends in health and ill-health and focused on issues of particular concern – in 1951 it was the increase in deaths from lung cancer and coronary heart disease. Cancer deaths are analysed in some detail and the report points to a trend in the literature that links them with cigarette smoking. It did not make specific recommendations save that further research was needed. The report is able to comment on the continuing success evident in a reduction in the incidence of infectious disease. It was an indication of this success that such diseases no longer dominated annual reports (by inference underlining the space this left for a consideration of chronic conditions).

Incidences of tuberculosis had fallen by 40 per cent in four years, although there were still 14,000 reported deaths each year. This particular battle had not yet been won. This was also the case with other infectious diseases where there had been a downturn in previous years but in 1951 some small increase – for example, deaths from whooping cough and measles had increased – and the report stressed that 'we must not relax the prophylactic measures which have brought about the major triumph' of the decrease in premature deaths from infectious disease.

Morbidity figures are acknowledged as of necessity less certain. But the report does identify and investigate incapacity – which it related to work absences and to medical consultancy rates. In turn these can be linked with specific occupational groups showing, for example, a low rate of consultation of doctors by agricultural workers and a high rate by workers in mines and quarries. Changes in nutrition, the impact of immunization campaigns and the progress of medical research are all reviewed.

In the realm of public health the report observes that the improvements in the general physical environment mean that people can enjoy a healthier and more agreeable life without having to make a great effort. There was a recognition that although the major benefits in public health might have been attributable to experts like sanitary technicians the major gains here had also been made and future improvements in public health might require a transfer of attention from the environment to the person.

Such annual reports provided Parliament with a picture of the current state of ill-health and with at least some of the more identifiable trends. In so doing they facilitated the opportunity for a more informed debate about health priorities. The reports included some specific policy recommendations; the 1951 report, for example, recommended increasing and improving pre-natal education. They also contained considerable guidance in abstracting from research a synopsis of current thinking; for example, in the 1951 report, on nutrition. In short, the reports provided useful material to inform a policy-making process susceptible to a rational approach to planning. Looked at from today these reports indicate trends that were becoming apparent and which still play central roles in policy-making, including the shift from a collectivist to an individual interpretation of preventive health and the recognition of the increased prominence of chronic disease.

The reports also offered research and advice that did not seem tied to a particular pressure group interest. The policy-making process is informed by research and by the expression of opinion from very many sources, but when your advice about nutrition comes from the British Sugar Council or when research into health is funded by tobacco companies or when you rely on doctors to evaluate and report on specific treatments in which they are involved the presence of an apparently independent body not tied to any pressure group, professional organization or political party appeared markedly useful. But as we have seen we cannot make the necessary first assumption about rationality!

Planning occurs within a particular action space and over time the space that is considered appropriate is modified. It certainly is limited. What is of central importance for what planners can offer is the definition of their acceptable authority and the scope of their remit. It could be argued that the most useful way to encourage good health would be to concentrate on income maintenance. It could also be argued that town planning and general environmental planning are starting points rather than peripheral concerns. The indivisibility of health ought to necessitate a central place for occupational health planning. But, as we have seen, the planning process is dominated by a medicalization of health and a politicization of priority setting, by expediency and by incrementalism. Instead of a straightforward model of action space one writer (Underwood 1976) has suggested that we seek to understand the planners 'potential, diffuse and debated action space'.

The formal process of planning in the NHS is a straightforward, legalistic and apparently rational process (Self 1977, p. 8) with a number of delineated aims, obligations and stages. These included a commitment to review all the alternatives, to identify and evaluate all the consequences that would arise from the pursuit of a particular policy and to assess how far one decision would accord with the overall plan developed in a district or region (Hunter 1980, p. 47). This is a recipe for perfection in a world not used to such achievements! Such an approach in practice is translated into a belief in the importance of seeking compromise and consensus and, as such, is in accord with the identified style of management practice before Griffiths.

To describe planning in such a rational way is to decontextualize it and, as such, render it meaningless in an environment where planning is about influence, politics and power. To pretend it is rational, or to pretend that consensus can be achieved and definitely should be sought, is to misconstrue the nature of the beast. But likewise the retreat to incremental, or decremental, responses to political and pressure group interaction is to suggest that, apart from at the margins, no real change is possible and that the notion of planning as involving future-orientated activity is a redundant one.

The argument develops, therefore, that planning does not exist. Whichever of the above stances it takes does not leave it without a role that can be understood as planning. But we said at the outset that planning might be simply defined as what planners do and I want to pause here and detail the process as it is understood by them. The operational process of planning has been summarized by Dunnell and Holland (1973, pp. 252–5) as consisting of seven stages:

1 Pre-planning, the assessment of the existing preconditions including existing legislation, administrative capacity, government commitment and intentions.
2 An identification of the ideal which represents the general political and social desires for change.
3 Setting objectives bearing in mind (1) and aiming as nearly as possible to achieve (2). This is a stage of assigning priorities and investigating the various ways of achieving them.
4 Drawing up the plan in terms of actual targets and the configuration of services that will emerge.
5 Resource allocation as a stage where labour, financial and capital resources are combined in the way most likely to achieve (4).
6 The establishment of a programme that combines (4) and (5) into an operational scheme.
7 A process of evaluation and reassessment questioning the extent to which objectives have been achieved and if results could have been better achieved using different means.

Such an ideal model should perhaps be countered immediately with two observations by less enamoured participants in the planning and decision-making process. The then Secretary of State, Norman Fowler, offered a reading of NHS history which said that 'interest groups believe the way to get more resources is to complain and keep on complaining and then more resources come' (*Panorama*, BBC Television, 17 October 1983). Certainly the ideal model misses out the role of pressure groups and the representation of interests by those outside the formal bureaucracy and machinery of government. It also does not recognize the power of bureaucratic maintenance and organizational inertia. An Australian report (Hospitals and Health Services Commission 1974, p. 228) commented on the amount of hospital resources that were needed and the arbitrariness of such decisions by saying that at any one time what was needed was what was available.

9 The Resource Allocation Working Party, Economics and Managerialism

There are three features characteristic of the present NHS that it is important to introduce into the analysis of the interaction of politics and planning. I will look at the issue of resource allocation and specifically at the Resource Allocation Working Party (RAWP). I will then look at attempts to introduce controls that would alter the place of clinical freedom in the planning of health care delivery. Finally, I will examine whether we should best replace the term 'planning' with 'management'. Does the post-Griffiths NHS manifest a new approach to deciding priorities?

RAWP is important for three reasons. First, its deliberations help in determining the amount of money allocated to different health regions and districts. Second, it has been consistent in NHS resource allocation since it was first applied to the budget of 1977–8 and as such presents an argument that planning does exist and is consistent over time, the initial report came out in 1976 (DHSS 1976a). Third, it represents a shift in funding from being based on activity levels, with allowances for growth and developments, to capitation-based finance with the objective of securing geographical equity in the availability of resources (Mays and Bevan 1987).

The report was produced in 14 months by an *ad hoc* group of NHS officers, DHSS Civil Servants and academics and it has survived almost unscathed, despite many criticisms, to the 1989 White Paper. Carrier (1978, p. 120) called RAWP 'the most significant attempt at a planned change in the NHS (notwithstanding the 1974 reorganization) since its inception in 1948'.

There had been a change in structure and an identification of the need to prioritize services for the mentally ill, handicapped and the elderly in 1974. In 1976 a new form of allocating funds was introduced. These have survived political changes and the turbulence of the years to remain as key factors in determining allocation policies and hence the operation and development of the NHS. The NHS may seem always to be undergoing change. When we look at the annual operational policies of health districts we can see considerable change brought about by alterations in short and medium term funding. But alongside this is a consistency over time in these major areas of priority and of funding rationale.

This consistency should not be interpreted as meaning that there was a close relationship between resource allocation and service planning. One suggestion has been that a split exists and this reflects a division within the DHSS (Butts *et al.* 1981, p. 42). In the DHSS groupings responsible for different activities could be identified. These, in turn, were linked with different groups outside the Department. The officials in policy groups were in close touch with pressure groups but not with the NHS management. In particular the professional advisory committees of doctors, nurses and midwives appeared to be lobbying to have shortcomings in services to particular client groups recognized and remedied. The results of these contacts were then seen by management as not having a real sense of the problems of running the NHS and reconciling different demands. This was exacerbated by the belief that the policy groups were not sensitive to the new demands imposed on managers of having to plan to a budget. There did not seem to be a group within the DHSS which could bring the sides together. The top officials appeared preoccupied with servicing the Minister in the sense of ensuring, or trying to ensure, that he was not vulnerable to political embarrassment. One manifestation of division was the apparent absence of co-ordination in what would appear intrinsically linked long-term objectives, geographic redistribution and redistribution by type of problem.

The division within the DHSS between planning and management was a long-standing one. Throughout the 1970s the Service Development Group worked separately from the Regional Group. Links between Service Development and Finance were tenuous and, when they did exist, seemed unconnected with the specific operations of RAWP. DHSS (1976a) considered itself concerned with the distribution of financial resources and not with how the regions should deploy these resources. RAWP was concerned with means and not ends (DHSS 1976a, para 1.5, p. 8). One hope entertained by the Griffiths reforms was that a management board would carry out that role of offering a clear strategic lead to the NHS and, in doing so, could reconcile planning and resource allocation. This has not happened, although it would appear that there is more sense of co-ordination than there was. But this has been achieved by the dominance of management, centrally controlled by resource allocations, and by target setting and not by progress in rational long-term planning.

There are three main areas of criticism of RAWP. First, its introduction underestimated the difficulties of moving to a new policy and away from the customary incremetalism. Second, the figures used to calculate the adjustments to funding under RAWP were clumsy. They measured only very limited aspects of health need and health delivery and generalized too districts and regions. In a region that appeared well off, and so ations restricted, there might be districts – or parts of much higher levels of need. (This is the argument that has been linked with the impact of RAWP on services in London.) Third, RAWP was introduced at a time when a number of other key changes were occurring, such as the introduction of cash limits, and there was not sufficient flexibility in the allocation of extra funding to ensure a reasonable transition to the new methods of allocation.

The assumption was that those areas which, under RAWP recommendations, received a restricted allocation would have to scrutinize all their services, particularly the more expensive specialist hospital services, to identify how they could continue to function with this restricted budget. The problem the health authorities encountered was doing this at a time of financial cutbacks and increasing demand.

Some of these criticisms were taken on by the DHSS when the NHS Management Board undertook a review of RAWP in 1986 (DHSS 1986b). Central to this review was the recognition of the problems in measuring morbidity and social deprivation (they were also concerned to review the problems created in cross-boundary flows, in teaching medical students and in the problems of the inner cities). RAWP used standardized mortality ratios in conjunction with figures on population size and age and sex structure. They were seeking a measure of need rather than of demand or of use. Relying on the latter might prompt a return to a model of incrementalism.

There have been many criticisms of such a basis for calculation (Mays and Bevan 1987, p. 148). Specifically it has been observed that the measures do not take into account morbidity that does not lead to death. But here there are two caveats. First, there is a strong correlation between morbidity, mortality and social deprivation. If an area is deprived, people will not just die earlier but will also get sick more. Second, no model has been proposed which will measure morbidity in a way that does not depend on supply of services. Any more suitable model would have to be very complex. For example, one might argue that the deprived areas have more need of resources because the infrastructure is such that they require more hospital care. Perhaps housing is not ideal for recuperative care, so that patients should stay in hospital longer. But the dynamic of that argument ought to lead to a questioning of housing policy and a realization that such a problem is not one the NHS, in the context of resource allocation, can reasonably solve. Any solution requires a recognition of the indivisibility of social policy. As I have argued earlier, to say that more is being spent on the NHS and at the same time to cut drastically money allocated to housing policy and to inhibit council repair budgets is to fail to understand that the nature of health need is more than the episodic treatment of illness.

As well as debates on the regional distribution of resources there have been developments leading to, and much discussion on, the introduction of devices that will allow more control over outputs within the service as opposed to the usual controls exercised, through funding, legislation and ministerial guidance, over inputs. Cash limits, performance indicators, the ubiquitous efficiency savings and discussion of clinical budgeting are the most important features to study. Some of these have figured many times in the previous presentation and I will only review the key points in this section.

I will begin by looking again at the attempt to apply economics to health care via the use of the Quality Adjusted Life Year (QALY). This links with discussions on clinical budgeting and is consistent with trends to introduce some curb on clinical freedom. As such it contains a challenge to many of the developed practices and enshrined customs of the NHS. The idea has been developed, in its present form, by Professor Alan Williams (1985). Williams describes his project as being concerned to associate real-world phenomena with particular concepts in a theoretical model and then to use that model, now with its interrelationships and implications, back in the real world of phenomena. In this case to use economics to help evaluate the outcome of various treatments possible under the NHS. But it is 'not just economics'; the model requires the ethical assumption that one year of healthy life expectancy is of equal value to everybody and that being dead is equally bad for everybody (Williams 1987, p. 565).

The ethics may be rudimentary, or fundamental, depending on how favourable you feel, but it is important to make them clear. In some of the ways the NHS has been seen to work, for example over the availability of kidney transplant and dialysis, the assumption seems to have been that some lives are more important than others. The service will be given to the young, to those providing for a family. Such decisions have been made as part of the general exercise of clinical freedom. Williams, at the very least, has done a considerable service in setting up the possibility for a more open discussion of these matters.

He is writing in a way that one would feel is consistent with many developments in contemporary policy-making and politics. One feature of the early years of the Thatcher government was that they were a time of some ascendancy for economists (Hearn and Small 1984). Undoubtedly there has also been evident an increase in concerns over costings and over efficiency, understood in an economic sense. But although such factors might be supposed to endear Professor Williams to policy-makers, there is another side to his work that they would find less appealing. There is a problem in asking people what they want, and in measuring outcome, in that you may in so doing create a demand that had been only latent. You risk disturbing not only professional power but bureaucratic inertia and political indifference.

General considerations aside Williams's work has been criticized in both its assumptions and its detail. For an economist the interesting feature of the NHS is that it provides an example of the distribution of scare resources to meet valued outcomes without the mediation of price to the patient. But it is a market not just without the price mechanism to the consumer. It is also a monopoly (private health care is not yet big enough to challenge this) where the producer is not only the sole supplier of goods but also tells consumers what they need and decides what will be produced. The opportunity economists see is to place into this neat system a real consideration of choice by the potential recipients of service, to replace the present professionally and politically defined priorities. In so doing Professor Williams is seeking to influence the practice of NHS managers and to add a further factor to the range of considerations employed by medical personnel, in particular consultants. He is aiming at two different constituencies which have been increasingly wary of each other. It is a wariness increased by the potential rise in managerial power consequent upon the general atmosphere of cost consciousness coming from the government and the structural and procedural changes emerging from the Griffiths reforms.

Williams (1985, p. 326) sums up his position in this way,

> The objective of economic appraisal is to ensure that as much benefit as possible is obtained from the resources devoted to health care. In principle the benefit is measured in terms of the effect on life expectancy adjusted for quality of life . . . [medical treatments] should be ranked so that activities that generate more gains to health for every pound of resources take priority over those that generate less; thus the general standard of health in the community would be correspondingly higher.

Contenders for additional resources should be compared, each time a decision on allocation of resources is made, to test which should be cut back and which expanded.

The QALY is identified using two criteria, disability and distress. Eight conditions of disability, ranging from no disability to unconscious, are combined with four levels of distress, from none to severe. A matrix can then be created with twenty-nine possible conditions. A sample population can then be asked to score various conditions, numerical scores can be aggregated and, indirectly, a community's valuation of the quality of life associated with various states of health can be arrived at. To move from this to QALY, a profile of what happens to a particular patient over time, after a specific medical treatment, is required. The next step is to move from the matrix, via the QALY, to include cost and then to construct a table of medical treatments in which it will be clear where resources can be directed to provide the greatest benefit for patients – on their own terms.

Williams has been criticized (Mulkay *et al.* 1987, p. 546) for 'imposing the discourse of economics upon the problems of NHS management and replacing their concerns with those of his own discipline'. But the model that exists, and to which Williams is writing in opposition, is one that also depends upon some problematical criteria. One measure that has been used is comparative rates of survival following interventions. But this ignores considerations about quality of life and shuts out treatments that are not primarily concerned with life and death issues. It elevates 'dramatic' medicine to an undeserved prominence (something that has happened throughout the history of hospital care). One commentator (Maynard 1986, p. 159) went further and suggested that the NHS suffers from 'the blinkered concerns of cost minimising accountants and benefit maximising clinicians'. Others have put it more crudely. The allocation of money is often about who shouts the loudest, and one very loud way to shout is by 'shroud waving' (*Safe in Our Hands*, BBC Radio 4, 20 August 1986). Ham (1981, p. 196) referred to this as 'planning by decibels'.

One criticism of the economists' approach to health planning is that it depoliticizes a profoundly political reality. It imposes its own rules of discourse and in so doing excludes some concerns from a legitimate place in the debate. Colin Thunhurst (1985–6, p. 25), suspicious of QALYs and still trying to work out exactly why, referred to the impact of cost–benefit analysis on the debate concerning the role of government in the late 1960s. The problem with cost–benefit analysis, he says, was that it took no account of 'externalities', the spin-off costs and benefits that follow particular decisions. For example, under the Beeching plan if a branch railway line cost more in upkeep than it took in ticket sales then it was closed down. But if there was no train then more money would have to be spent on the upkeep of roads in the area, there would be more pollution and more traffic accidents. Cost–benefit analysis may try to 'internalise the externalities' but can only do so by giving them a monetary value and some of them may not be readily convertible into this 'currency'. Besides not all may be considered. Thunhurst's is a persuasive position. To present an economic discourse instead of a medical one is not to empower the potential consumer but rather to replace one system of dominance with another. There are parallels in changes in laws relating to abortion. Here there was a limited shift of power from the law to medicine but not to a woman's right to choose (Bland 1985).

But we need to ask once more what the alternative is. In the past problems were medicalized and the dominant sphere was a scientific one. Such discourse is also depoliticizing, exclusive and excluding. We are in a by now familiar dilemma. Are we seeking to set up better structures? If so, the arrival of economists can be understood as at least one move towards opening up debate. Or are we looking for an ideal? If so, QALY and the march of the economists is not it!

In its attempts to develop a more efficient use of resources the government introduced performance indicators following the Duthie Report (DHSS 1981). This report had compared the sizes of waiting lists for orthopaedic services between regions. It prompted a review of ways that information could be assembled to enable a manager to assess the efficiency of a service for which he or she was responsible. Underlying this concern was a belief that the NHS could, and should, provide a better service using the resources currently available to it. This links with the consideration of the place of efficiency savings. If the service could perform better with a given level of resource then some of that resource may be diverted to other purposes. The government then includes this diverted resource as representing an increase in funding. Figures for anticipated efficiency savings are built into NHS financial programmes accordingly.

Performance indicators have to be seen alongside the introduction of new management practices and specifically managerial accountability. They are an attempt to introduce more central control of expenditure and more effective scrutiny of performance. The spur to such changes was not just the general increase in centralized power evident in the NHS since 1979 but, specifically, a criticism from the House of Commons Committee of Public Accounts (1981). This reported a lack of effective control over those financial matters that had been delegated to regional health authorities. The Committee acknowledged that the DHSS could not control everything but that performance indicators, set centrally, could be an effective means of furthering such control as was possible.

> The purpose of the Performance Indicator package was to provide managers with useful information about the use of resources at District level in a systematic fashion, set within a national framework to enable comparisons to be made with other Districts. This information was supplemented with values for Regional and National averages (Allen *et al.* 1987, p. 72).

A trial run was carried out in the Northern region and then the first set of national figures was introduced for use by the district health authorities in September 1983. They covered the areas of manpower, finance, ambulance services, estate management and clinical activity. The clinical activity section was divided into specialisms: general medicine, general surgery, gynaecology, obstetrics and trauma and orthopaedic surgery. The resulting figures were presented in such a way as to allow districts to see relative levels of activity and cost in other districts. If they were a league table, and the government were at pains to say they were not, then they were a league table without considerations of health outcomes or the quality of care. A study of the use of performance indicators in three districts by Allen *et al.* found that the region used them to set targets for improvements and evaluate success in areas such as throughput in hospitals and the achievement of specific staffing levels. Districts had to report performance in annual reviews and regions would follow up to ask why targets had not been met. Both for planning staff and management the change that resulted was significant. The introduction of detailed scrutiny and consequent accountability was something that had not previously been perceived as central to the planning process.

There have been numerous criticisms of the use of performance indicators, the first of which is that they do not measure performance. They may be based on admission rates, average length of stay, annual throughput per bed, turnover interval, cost per day, or ratio of trained to untrained staff, and, as such, they measure some inputs. But they say nothing about performance in terms of the impact on the health status of the population the district serves. A second criticism is that they do not compare like with like in that hospitals, and indeed health districts, operate in environments where there are different levels of need and of demand. A third criticism is that there is a problem in assembling accurate data on which to base performance indicators. Allen *et al.*'s study found data suspect in terms of its not being comprehensive or topical. It was often poorly recorded and calculated. They concluded that the districts studied believed that it was 'statistics which are in need of improvement rather than performance' (Allen *et al.* 1987, p. 79). Further, it is argued that even if the indicators were accurate there would be variations from one district to another because of random factors. As such, districts argue, it would be better to consider major shortfalls in performance rather than marginal variations. The very detail of the method undermines its validity.

With the exception of the first criticism, it would appear that refining the method of collection and calculation would remove many of the objections. But the question remains whether all the effort in assembling the figures is worth it! There are some arguments that the existence of performance indicators helps provide 'a useful index of suspicion' (Parker, quoted in Allen *et al.* 1987, p. 82) and a 'powerful tool if they are used in sets as they have the ability to tip the balance in favour of action, whereas without their assistance no action may be taken' (Yates, quoted in Allen *et al.* 1987, p. 82). But, if this is the way they can be of help, their detrimental impact is of more concern. Such a reductionist model of understanding planning need risks managers deciding that they have to achieve the norm whether to do so is efficient in terms of the needs of their districts or not.

Performance indicators were being introduced at a time when the cash-limits policy was continuing and, as such, this underlines the importance of seeking to understand all these central controls in terms of their cumulative impact on health planning and the scope for local initiative. To assess the cash-limits policy I will refer to a 1983 DHSS Health Circular

((83)16). Any health circular deserves close review in terms of the language it uses and the impact it is likely to have on regions and districts. Like its predecessors, and those that followed it, the Circular passes on resource planning assumptions but reminds those receiving the Circular that they should plan flexibly because the annual review of public expenditure had not yet been issued and it might necessitate 'variations above or below the planning assumptions'. It goes on to say that 'the first obligation upon Authorities is to comply with their statutory duty not to exceed their cash limits'. To this end all expenditure should be reviewed. There should be a renewed drive to achieve economies and to reduce costs, particularly in the case of less essential expenditure on goods and services, and there needs to be better control of NHS manpower. Such language underlines two things. The first is that the regions and districts were being asked to plan but were not being given the security to do so. To say that you cannot assume that resource figures are reliable is to undermine any detailed planning and to provoke safety-first decision-making that does not run the risk of over-commitment.

The second feature of this approach is its emphasis on not exceeding cash limits. If this is the first obligation of authorities, what has happened to the obligation to meet the health needs and treat the ill-health of the locality served? This is not just semantics but an important part of the project of creating, or maintaining, a paradigm of planning that elevates input above outputs. It produces the kinds of response from planners and managers, all aware of the degree of scrutiny within the system, that makes them more concerned with the league table of performance indicators than with the provision of a balanced service for their district or with the levels of morbidity there apparent.

The extent of central control and the extension of this into manpower levels was also evident in this Circular. There had been, in 1982 and 1983 Health Circulars ((82)14; (83)4) that had asked regions to submit to the DHSS manpower targets for March 1984. But 'progress has fallen short of what is desired and expected' and ministers had now decided that manpower control needed to be improved as a matter of urgency. The intention was to achieve firm targets and the DHSS gave 'indicative figures' to be achieved by 31 March 1984 of a reduction of 0.75–1 per cent in overall staff numbers from the total employed at 31 March 1983. Within these figures posts other than doctors, dentists, nurses, midwives, technical and professional staff were expected to reduce more sharply, by 1.35–1.8 per cent. No vacancy should be filled unless there was a clear case for its continuation; the health authority was expected to ensure that there was a service justification for every post created. Progress towards targets would be monitored using the quarterly manpower counts and would be included in the regional review process. (One interesting feature of a study of such Health Circulars is that they present a clear picture of intentions that is in contrast to the obfuscation of the parliamentary answer or the ministerial speech.)

It might be argued that, in themselves, such directives have some things that would have been consistent over time. Health authorities would presumably say that they always had service justification for appointing people and that vacancies were filled because they were 'real jobs' and needed to be carried out. But in the past there were not such closely scrutinized cash limits (cash limits had been in force since introduced by the Labour government in 1976) and manpower targets. Indeed the cuts in manpower being considered in Health Circular (83)16 were considerable. But the further dimension here was that this was the time when the Griffiths Report (DHSS 1983a) was criticizing consensus management (the Griffiths Report came out in October, this Circular was from August) and there were calls for the establishment of the Rayner scrutinies – initially into the costs of non-ambulance transport and NHS recruitment. Taken together, these were to provide a continuing machinery of scrutiny. In themselves each of these developments was important, but seen cumulatively they marked a significant change in the custom and practice of the NHS.

Rayner was brought in to advise the government in 1979 and the approach bearing his name was first applied in 1982. The method was to introduce short intensive scrutiny of specific areas by officers from within the NHS. A number of areas were subjected to such scrutiny. Some of the reports were controversial – the proposal to save up to £750 million by selling NHS property, for example. Others identified what had been long-running problems in effective administration – the collection of payments due to health authorities under the provision of the Road Traffic Act was one such area. By 1984 the DHSS was being asked to take action on a number of the Rayner scrutinies and to report the savings achieved as a result to the DHSS. Griffiths was from Sainsbury's and Lord Rayner from Marks and Spencer; this was the era of the grocer.

In 1983 policy on competitive tendering was set out in Health Circular (83)18. Authorities were asked to test the cost effectiveness of catering, domestic and laundry services by inviting tenders for the provision of these services from their own staff and from outside contractors. DHAs were requested to submit a timetable for competitive tendering to enable tenders for all services to be submitted by September 1986 (Ham 1985, pp. 48–9). We have seen on pages 99–100 the impact of this in terms of the number of contracts given to external tenders.

I am not so concerned with the detail of all these changes in this chapter but rather to present them as part of a cumulative process by which the regions and districts were subject to an increasing measure of detailed direction from the centre. Two more relevant points are, first, that Griffiths reforms meant that the newly appointed general managers and indeed the whole of the management structure at the top of each unit were to be subject to scrutiny, to a measure of payment by results and to the possibility of removal from office at the point of contract renewal if they had not satisfied the identified requirements of the post. Who decided these requirements? The DHSS and the Secretary of State, advised by regions and by district chairmen. Second, the allocation of funds was tied to a calculation of efficiency savings that also set imperatives in terms of management and planning policy. Planning to satisfy the centre might accord with the specifics of local need but, if it did, it would be more by good fortune than conscious design.

To finish this chapter I want to make some brief concluding remarks on the nature of the relationship between planning and management and how they developed under the Conservative government after 1979. But, as with all these things, one has to begin a little further back.

The 1974 reorganization, presented to Parliament by Sir Keith Joseph, was an explicit attempt to introduce the ideas of responsible managerialism. The agenda Sir Keith had identified was one of a need to increase efficiency, and the way to this was through management, the combination of the development of managerial expertise and corporate accountability. The Labour government which had been in office until 1970, and its Secretary of State, Richard Crossman, had believed in responsiveness and representation as being more important paradigms. Such an approach would contribute to a better, more efficient, service (but with efficiency measured in terms of appropriateness not cost).

If the political parties differed it did appear that from the late 1960s the argument in the DHSS had been won. The better use of resources and the development of detailed and efficient management were seen as two sides of the same coin. This was translated into the reform proposals and became a commitment by Sir Keith Joseph on which he was not prepared to waver.

But it was not just that the arrival of managerialism came from the commitment of Sir Keith Joseph. There was also evident a general trend within conservatism and within the country. Specifically in regard to the NHS there had been a development of such ideas from the 1960s. The Salmon Report (Ministry of Health, 1966) was a managerial reform of nursing (Brian Salmon, who chaired this report on the organization of nursing services, was a businessman from Lyons, the food distributors). It was undertaken in an atmosphere where the importance of efficiency was a characteristic very evident in the rhetoric of the Wilson style of Labourism and of Heath's Conservatism.

There were then the Cogwheel Reports (Ministry of Health 1967; DHSS 1972; 1974) on the organization of medical staff and the contributions of medicine to policy-making. They were called Cogwheel because of the design on the cover, not because there was a grocer called Cogwheel on the committee! The Farquaharson-Lang Report (DHSS 1974) on the administrative practices of hospital authorities informed the production of the 'Grey Book' on 'Management Arrangements for the Reorganised NHS'. This set out in some detail the functions of each tier of the structure of the NHS and provided job descriptions for health authority officers.

The dominant approach became one based on the establishment of teamwork without hierarchy, controlled through collective responsibility. The aim was the establishment of a health service that could achieve both greater efficiency and be responsive to the government's aims. Consensus management by management teams in each authority, both region and area, would be the pattern. Teams were to be made up of the major professional groupings: the administrator; the treasurer; the nursing officer; the community physician; two elected medical representatives; a consultant from the Medical Executive Committee and a GP. At region and at area the so-constituted management team was responsible to an appointed body of health authority members. It was intended that these members, and the chairmen of the authority, would concentrate on general policy-making and monitoring performance while the management team had an executive role. Management would also service the members and would be responsible for the production of the authority's plan. At district level the management team (DMT) was collectively responsible for keeping district services under review and implementing area policies.

This development of managerialism went alongside the belief in the rationality of the planning process and both appeared, or were presented, as complementary developments to make the system work more effectively and more in accord with the nationally decided aims and objectives. Planning was seen, by the 1974 reorganization, as being the single most important influence for better resource allocation. It was to be a way of achieving a national strategy of objectives, standards and priorities (Allsop 1984, p. 66). There was to be a national system that was comprehensive in terms of service provision and involved co-operation with local authority social services departments via joint consultative committes (JCCs) and the public via community health councils. There were to be both long and short term planning cycles, the strategic and operational plans. Guidelines on policy were to be passed down from the DHSS to the region and then to the area. But the actual preparation of the plan was to begin at district level, the level closest to service delivery. There were to be joint care planning teams at district levels that included GPs and representatives of social services departments. These would be organized around identified-need groups like the elderly or the mentally handicapped. They would produce information about existing provision and make proposals for change. JCCs at area level were to have planning teams to look at particular groups and their needs.

This approach, placing management and planning close together and in harmony, was argued as something non-contentious, almost non-political. It might be that the ends sought, or the results achieved, would excite controversy, but the means, it was assumed, should be accepted by all reasonable and concerned people.

It is apposite here to reflect on the general tenor of ideological discussion in the Conservative Party and on the Right in general. In the years immediately before 1979 and in the early days of Mrs Thatcher's first term in government there was evident an important ideological shift towards monetarism and towards ideas critical of economic planning in general. It was a time when F.A. von Hayek's work, most notably *The Road to Serfdom* (Hayek 1944), was gaining many adherents in the Conservative Party. It is important to note because it helps locate the discussions about management and planning in the context of the developing ideology and the dominant form of discourse in terms of the role of the state in society.

Hayek had argued that central economic planning led inescapably to totalitarianism: 'Planning of any kind . . . was an offence against nature, a vastly presumptuous and self defeating attempt to impose on the myriad wishes and habits of men and women a single scheme of organisation' (Hugo Young, in the Guardian, 8 October 1984, 'celebrating' the fortieth anniversary of the publication of *The Road to Serfdom*). Hayek argues that monopolies are safer in private than in public hands and that social welfare spending should be merely the residual of economic policy. The very existence of such a concept as social justice is questioned. There cannot be a combination of both freedom and planning. This position represented a major challenge to the post-war consensus which was built on the continuation of wartime interventionism and planning into the peacetime life of the United Kingdom and was most clearly exemplified in the welfare state.

Hayek's contribution to the new conservatism was important, as was that of Friedman, and I have reviewed the work of Niskanen in an earlier chapter. But there remains the apparent paradox inherent in attempts to operationalize such ideas. In seeking to withdraw from some areas there appears to develop a need to intervene more dramatically in others. There is a bifurcation of state activity. In the area covered by the DHSS an apparent wish to reduce the role of the government exists at the same time as managerial and planning systems are developed that appear to increase the effective element of central direction. In terms of spending, a determined ideology committed to its reduction in fact spends at record levels and then seeks, at least in regard to the NHS, to claim credit for this. Such theory–practice dichotomies are very intricate!

10   General Management

The introduction of general management was predicated on a belief that the commercial sector had skills that would enhance the management performance of the NHS. It was assumed that private sector management had to be effective or it would not survive, but that effectiveness was not solely related to the generation of profit. Indeed the assumption seemed to be that 'many aspects of management are universally applicable, and merely sharpened by the profit motive' (Arnold 1987, p. 332). Davidson (1987) has identified the 'new managerialism' as something that began to take hold of the NHS at the start of the 1980s; by 1982

> management and managerial preoccupations took over the NHS and began to set the parameters within which we now think about public health care...Management ideas now provide the dominant intellectual framework within which the health service thinks about itself and its role in society.

He argues that, in itself, management did not of necessity mean a pre-occupation with 'narrow issues of administrative efficiency'. But the great store set on performance indicators and measurable activity in themselves structured and dominated the new management ideology and practice. It was the coexistence of a wish to make the NHS more akin, managerially, to the private sector with a wish to exercise more direct and effective central control that explains why this particular form became dominant.

If there was an assumption about the transferability of skills and practices there were also evident some features of the NHS that appeared to be specific to it. Most notable of these were the extent of political considerations in the process of planning and of management and the presence of a countervailing power base in medicine.

The management ideas that the government was assuming should present a paradigm for NHS practice were only one model of private sector management and a model not at the forefront of creative thinking in management study.

> Management thinking increasingly stresses the breaking down of the old relationship as organisations adopt more fluid responsive structures and as individuals seek greater job satisfaction, more freedom and high levels of performance (Arnold 1987, p. 332).

If Davidson is correct the NHS is certainly not pursuing these kinds of structure and practice. In this chapter I want, simply, to look at one example of the ideas current in the private sector and relate them to the specifics of the NHS, and thus seek similarities and differences. I will then look at the experience of 'outsiders' who have joined NHS management teams as general managers and comment on their encounter with the particular conditions noted above.

Sir John Harvey-Jones's (1988) reflections on his leadership of ICI, the United Kingdom's largest manufacturing company, are revealing even in their title, *Making It Happen*. The top job, he tells us, possesses almost limitless opportunity to be ineffective! His advice is to be totally clear about how you are going to set about it. There are non-executive and executive activities. The former are concerned with the management of the actual board, and the external environment, as well as ensuring that mechanisms are in place to develop strategies and clear policies on the many issues on which the board has responsibility. The latter has the responsibility for seeing that the policies are carried out and managing that process. Harvey-Jones qualifies this scope for the leader with a realization that the company has already been moving in one direction, it has a number of employees in particular places and it has a sense of values. He also discusses the realization that if you are involved internationally then it is essential to be aware of differences:

> Americans use language in a different way, they are motivated by different things . . . they apply a different perspective of history, and they are the prisoners of different perspectives from ourselves.

Or, on the subject of work in India:

> Indian people love to talk, discuss, examine, debate. The short, crisp discussion and decision makes them feel uncomfortable. They do not feel that the many ramifications that they would wish to pursue have been properly explored.

If we transpose Harvey-Jones's thoughts to the NHS we see in the management practice therein some of the same kinds of structure and problem. We need only to change the discussion about international differences to one of professional differences. The introduction of general management into the NHS set up the possibility of a clash of occupational cultures. Clashes had occurred before but had not been among equals. The dominance of medicine was now to be challenged. It also highlighted the paradox between central control and managerial accountability.

Harvey-Jones saw a difference in the development of strategy and policy, on the one hand, and the need to ensure that policies are carried out, on the other. In some commercial organizations that 'top' job is divided (not in ICI); in the NHS it is confused!

I have looked, in earlier chapters, at the impact of general management in the DHSS and the evident conflicts displayed so graphically in the appointment and then resignation of Victor Paige as chairman of the NHS Management Board. By mid-July 1987, 13 general managers had left, or were in the process of leaving, before the end of their contract (or their contract was not being renewed). Four of these had been appointed as general managers directly from other NHS posts, nine were 'outsiders' (six from the private sector and three from the armed forces). Not all had left because of problems in the job; some had moved to obtain promotion. But it was from the ranks of the outsiders that those who had left because of irreconcilable differences had come. Sometimes their departures were accompanied by considerable publicity and evident rancour (Alleway 1987).

As the newly created vacancies consequent upon their departure were filled none of the posts went to an industrialist or a businessman. Three authorities had, by September 1987, still to appoint, six jobs had gone to NHS employees, one to a director of social services (Andrew Foster, moving from North Yorkshire to be General Manager of Yorkshire RHA), one to a former NHS administrator who had private sector experience and two to members of the armed forces.

The drop-out rate was small, about 5 per cent of all general managers. But the reasons outsiders left are interesting, not least in what they indicate about the problems of joining the NHS and the differences either with expectations or with the usefulness of previous experiences. The NHS Management Board's Chief Executive, Len Peach, attributed the higher drop-out rate among outsiders to four factors. First, some were not good enough. Second, some received inadequate help from chairmen, authorities and local managers. Third, some were not ready for the immense culture shock joining the NHS involved. Fourth, some were not equipped with the skills to succeed in the 'goldfish bowl atmosphere' of an organization operating in the political arena. Peach looked forward to a solution that saw the NHS drawing on internal talent and expected that 'within the next few years the NHS will no longer need to look outside the service to find its managers . . . Everything I have seen indicates that the talent in the service is as good as any you can find outside' (*Health and Social Services Journal*, 16 July 1987, p. 818). With this recognition we have moved considerably far from the implied criticism of the standard of management and the capacity for people in post to adapt in the ways required inherent in the Griffiths Report.

We will be better equipped to understand the early years of general management from the point of view of the managers as a two-year research project, the Templeton Study, continues to make known its findings. One preoccupation this project has described is that of the relationship between managers and doctors. Managers see the need for, and difficulty of, involving clinicians in management. Two quotes illustrate some of the difficulties perceived by managers:

> The doctors lead the technology and therefore the pattern of the service. Unless managers get the doctors with them, everything else is just window dressing. That is where you have to get change ... The glorious Griffiths image of the District General Manager cutting through the bureaucratic undergrowth is just hogwash. You can cut through it as much as you like, but when you have done it you are just left there up against the consultants who are just saying 'no' (Gabbay and Dopson 1987, p. 1042).

What is being identified in the Templeton Study is not just differences in power but also in language and understanding (concerns not far different from those of Harvey-Jones and the problems of multinationals). Gabbay and Dopson (1987) sum up by saying that:

> Medical training stresses personal prowess in the achievement of short term goals for individual patients, regardless of cost. Managers are trained to stress the virtues of developing interpersonal and other skills so as to contribute as members of an organisation, and to make optimum use of limited resources while working towards long term goals.

Even the style of expression of doctors and managers differs. Gabbay and Dopson (1987) describe the former as having conversations that might be heard by non-doctors as brusque, direct and harsh, while the latter are described as elliptical, woolly and evasive. These descriptions of different styles should be seen in the context of doctors' fears about clinical freedom in an NHS. They stress the danger of managerial powers (real or threatened) like clinical evaluation. To this must be added for managers, short-term fixed contracts, payment by results and appointment and accountability upwards to the Minister, with a consequent sense of urgency and insecurity. The result is a perception by some consultants that the manager is just there to impose centrally decided constraints. Words and phrases that managers use like 'quality assurance', 'performance review', 'objective setting', 'monitoring' and 'efficiency' may sound different to those consultants who feel they all resonate with the voice of central control. Likewise, managers may see clinicians as anachronistic reactionaries unable to see either the common good or the nature of contemporary political and economic change.

The dilemmas in creating interoccupational relationships in a situation rife with so many structural and ideological differences are considerable. But some progress does appear to have been made. The Templeton Study discusses the need to identify the managerial things clinicians do anyway. 'Doctors make management decisions about the short term allocation of resources for individual patients. Managers must make long term decisions in order to meet the changing needs of the community' (Gabbay and Dopson 1987, p. 1043). Balancing the short and long term becomes the focus for the frustrations and tensions evident in the system. It is, of course, not enough to seek a resolution by convincing doctors that management is not something to be feared as it is the same as something they have been doing anyway. But it is a start. The parts of the NHS cannot be seen separately from the whole. The whole has to include the organization, the politics, the history and the ideology. Just as one cannot look to management to explain the shortcomings of the system one cannot look to modified management to put it all right.

Prevalent in both political and planning talk in the NHS is a construct of 'business management'. There is a belief that what has been good for business would be good for the NHS. This is manifest in everything from the choice of persons to head inquiries to the language of 'efficiency' and to the selection of managers. I want now to question two things: first, the assumption of transferability from business to the NHS; and second, whether in so seeking to impose this model there has been a misunderstanding of what is 'good for business' and specifically the relationship between planning and business.

Michael Porter of the Harvard Business School, writing in *The Economist*, presents a very useful history, critique and reformulation of the place of strategic planning and attempts to convert it into 'the vital management discipline it needs to be' (Porter 1987, p. 21). Strategic planning was born in a flurry of optimism and industrial growth in the 1960s and early 1970s, he says. Every business aspired to having a strategic planning staff and every business school had a planning curriculum. But by the 1980s the 'fashion' had shifted. The new buzz words were 'corporate culture', 'quality' and 'implementation'. Japanese companies, it was observed, did not prepare corporate plans. Porter recognizes that the criticism of strategic planning was well deserved in that such planning had not, in most companies, contributed to strategic thinking.

Strategic planning grew out of two streams of thinking about management practice. The first was linked with a shift from annual budgets to five-year plans because of a recognition that the financial consequences of decisions were often long-term. Porter links this with a post-Second World War move to install formal budgeting as a device to improve control of operations in a business. The second, pioneered, he says, at Harvard, was the school of thought that highlighted the importance of having an overall corporate strategy. Companies might have had one of these but they had remained largely intuitive and implicit. Management theory had concentrated on parts – like production, finance, marketing, logistics, and so on. In the 1960s it was this approach that was supplemented with formal planning systems. Planning guidelines were issued and financial projections appeared everywhere. Corporate planners became the new key personnel. They 'drafted guidelines, set schedules, cajoled line managers and coached top executives in carrying out the planning process' (Porter 1987, p. 21). Many managers were unfamiliar with this new discipline and found it hard, without detailed guidance, to know what constituted strategic thinking. Porter uses the example of General Electric to illustrate some of the problems and, as I summarize them, it is possible to see parallels with the NHS.

Planning in diversified firms faced serious problems of what businesses to compete in and how to allocate resources among the constituent parts. For General Electric the problem was even more complex because all those parts necessitated considerable capital investment. Not all needs could be met but deciding priorities was difficult. In theory top managers had the power to make allocation decisions but they did not have the knowledge to permit them to exercise this power. That knowledge was locked up in the parts of the company. 'Skilful company executives, with facile answers to every head office question, obtained finance because the conglomerate's managers had little ammunition with which to deny their requests' (Porter 1987, p. 21).

What followed the discovery of such processes was advice, often from the growing number of strategic consultancy firms, on ways of moving ahead with strategy and not being dominated by sectional interests or by the exigencies of day-to-day business life. Much of this advice seemed to be dependent on the creation and utilization of a model that would permit the comparison of disparate activities. Examples of such models included calculating relative market share for each part of the company's activities and investing in those areas where the figure was larger. The assumption was that the company with the largest cumulative volume in any one sector would have the lowest cost and so it would make the company more competitive, and profitable, to seek such sectoral pre-eminence. Other models, like this one, were simplistic and mechanistic and their failure precipitated an attack on planning which achieved considerable momentum by the mid-1980s (at the time when the NHS was becoming even more committed to it).

The attack on planning was varied. There was a growing recognition that strategic planning was not producing strategic thinking:

> Instead of clarifying and communicating strategy, the outcome of laborious strategic planning exercises was thick binders which had little, if any, impact on action. Form dominated substance. Meaningless long term projections obscured strategic insight. Strategic planners had captured the process, filling out plans which were reviewed by yet other planners. Line managers tolerated planning, but increasingly dismissed it as irrelevant ritual (Porter 1987, p. 22).

Strategic planning models based on a dominant single variable (whatever it was) encountered serious problems in achieving the objective hoped for.

Then came the Japanese. Their success was identified not with planning but with a concentration on quality, productivity and teamwork. New themes emerging included an emphasis on corporate culture and on entrepreneurship or, as Porter called it, 'intrapreneurship' – and these people did not need to fill out strategic plans. 'It had suddenly become embarrassing to talk about strategic planning. Some companies went so far as to dismantle their planning process altogether, sometimes with a relish that belied years of frustration' (Porter 1987, p. 22).

Porter is not arguing for the end of planning but for its revitalization. Strategy cannot be separated from implementation and it cannot occur only once a year. He argues that it should become the job of line managers, not of head office staff. The best systems will be where representatives from different parts of an organization can meet together, under the leadership of a general manager, to debate and resolve the trade-offs that will be required. The planner's role should shift from that of doer to that of facilitator and integrator.

> Good strategic thinking requires fewer planning guidelines. It requires the recognition that planning is just one part of a complex of concerns that includes, amongst other things, quality and corporate culture. It is no good having one of these if the others are not in harmony with it. One cannot ignore quality no matter how elegant is the strategic plan (Porter 1987, p. 27).

These observations by Porter are indicative of a considerable debate within management and business studies. They highlight conflicting thoughts that have emerged from both theorizing about management and from the evaluation of different practices. What is most important for our study of the NHS is, first, a recognition of the shortcomings of the imposed and separate strategic plan; and second, a realization that there is no single planning orthodoxy. Politicians and the Press appear to assume that there is a common understanding of what management and planning ideally is. These are not uncontested constructs.

The enthusiasm for managerialism might be a long-standing one but it has to be located in the context of an emphasis on the control of public expenditure. It may be that managerialism is viewed as a euphemism for economizing – things are not always what they seem!

Sir Keith Joseph's managerialism was not developed with such a narrow cost imperative. There may have been a cost dimension but the sort of central control he was seeking through the changes he introduced was concerned with compliance with policy as well as cost directives. The Joseph changes saw a service in which chief officers would manage and authorities would supervise and oversee (House of Commons 1972, para. 93). Managerial relations would be characterized by delegation downwards matched by accountability upwards.

One senses in such a hierarchical system that the word used may be 'management' but the skills required are those of an administrator. It is as if the wish is to call someone a manager so that he or she can be called to task should objectives not be met but not give him or her much scope for independent manoeuvre.

In much of the literature on the organization of business a distinction is drawn between management, administration and policy-making. A good manager is, according to one American source (Wrapp 1967), someone who is

> able to move his organisation significantly towards the goals he has set, whether measured by higher return on investment, product improvement, development or management talent, faster growth in sales and earnings, or some other standard.

The role is essentially a dynamic one and contrasts with that of the administrator whose role is principally to maintain the status quo.

> Keeping the wheels turning in a direction already set is a relatively simple task, compared to that of directing the introduction of a continuing flow of changes and innovations, and preventing the organisation from flying apart under the pressure (Wrapp 1967, p. 93).

This leaves out policy considerations; good managers do not involve themselves with this, according to Wrapp. It is a mistake to equate well-defined policies and objectives with good management. Decisions are best made not in a rational comprehensive way in which, in response to each issue, the decision-maker proceeds deliberately, one step at a time, to collect complete data, to analyse them thoroughly, to study a wide range of alternatives, and finally to formulate a detailed course of action. Rather decisions are best made according to a method of 'successive limited comparison' in which decision-makers compare alternatives open to them in order to learn which most closely approximates to the objectives in mind. This is essentially best understood not as a rational but as an opportunistic approach, 'the manager as a muddler but a muddler with a purpose' (Lindblom 1964). A similar notion is that of the 'cascade approach' which envisages

> the generation of rules for problem solution and then their successive refinement over time as a solution to particular problems is attempted. This process gives the impression of solving a problem several times over but with successively more precise results (Ansoff 1965).

Viewing management in these terms helps in understanding the NHS. It points to the places management can easily fit and the areas of possible dislocation and difficulty. Overtly there would appear to be an area of experience – identified as incrementalism – where such models seem appropriate. If much decision-making and planning in health is dominated by servicing what is, as opposed to planning for what might be, then successive limited comparisons would seem both a useful and realistic model for management to adopt. Likewise, the cascade approach fits well with the idea of a manager having to harmonize the efforts of disparate occupational and interest groups around compromise formations that evolve over time. These models allow for the separation of policy-making and planning, although here they do leave us the question of what planning is in such an organizational structure. We are also left with the need to examine missing factors such as power, conflict and accountability.

PART IV

Conclusions

11 Conclusions

As I write this conclusion, in March 1989, it is possible to examine the events of recent months to ascertain how far they have conformed with the identified themes of this work. I know this is a move that has shades of Sisyphus – all writers and researchers know there has to be a point where you say enough and no more – but in this case a brief résumé of the intervening months does provide possibilities that I will seek to exploit.

In my detailed review of the health system in both the public and private sphere of policy-making I identified a number of areas of concern: planning, privatization, finance (in particular, cuts in provision), and a number of determining trends. These have been the conflict between medicine and management as dominant paradigms; the shift towards the public sphere as ideological and structural changes posed problems for the established forms of pressure group influence; the continuing preoccupation with a politics of presentation most exemplified by the debate over 'real' spending figures; the wish to maintain an effective interventionist state while encouraging a diminution of its direct ownership (the bifurcation of control and ownership); the relationship between the welfare state as an ideological construct designed to both deliver welfare and confer legitimacy and the attempt to reconstruct this in favour of something 'earned'.

In this short chapter I will attempt to bring up to date the detailed examination of the operation of politics and planning in health. There is evident a continuity of concern and all the previously identified areas are once more present.

Two of the major concerns of the period to be examined have been the government's instigation of an inquiry into the NHS and the changes in the structure and conditions of service of nurses and midwives. Both have a relevance in examinations of the relative importance of professional and managerial power in the NHS. The inquiry was set up in a way that suggested that a primary function it would serve would be to head off criticism that the government had faced, particularly from its own supporters. It read like a device to gain time and also to offer a way out for back-benchers critical of the detail of policy. There was no indication that the inquiry would seek widespread consultation and hence no likelihood that it would come up with ideas critical of the general stance of the government.

It would have been possible to set up a Royal Commission with a membership reflecting a range of opinion and a range of interested parties. But Royal Commissions have, as Hugo Young noted in the *Guardian* (9 February 1988), 'been consigned by Mrs Thatcher to the museum of consensual antiquities'. Nor was the inquiry to be carried out by a small team of respected outsiders; 'the Government believes there is no such thing as apolitical knowledge . . . experts . . . are merely politicians flying under bogus colours'. An inquiry team was constituted of the government's own experts. As such it offered a means of examining ways the current direction of change in the NHS could be better facilitated, 'better' meaning with less cost politically and economically. It also served as a location from which could come ideas pushing at the edges of the current consensus, ideas such as the further introduction of the market into health (see Association of Community Health Councils 1988). Junior ministers, including those like Christopher Chope who, as leader of Wandsworth Council, had acted in a way that tested the limits of Thatcherism in local government, were invited to give their opinions to Mrs Thatcher directly. Testing the limits of the possible by leaks is a well-tried method and has the added advantage of making subsequent policy intentions appear 'not so bad' (at least they didn't . . .!).

As finally constituted, the Health Review Committee was made up of a small group of Cabinet ministers and was chaired by the Prime Minister. Perhaps the most important event during its deliberations was the change in organizational structure and personnel in July 1988 which saw the DHSS divided and a separate Ministry of Health set up with Kenneth Clarke at its head. The Committee, the Chancellor of the Exchequer, Nigel Lawson, the Chief Secretary to the Treasury, John Major, were there throughout, with John Moore and Tony Newton from the DHSS replaced by Clarke. Peter Walker and Malcolm Rifkind (representing Wales and Scotland) were concerned to effect real changes while minimizing the risk of political damage. The more overtly radical recommendations were diverted into the final 'internal market' proposals which we might call radicalism by stealth.

The White Paper that resulted from these deliberations, *Working for Patients* (Department of Health 1989) is presented, in the Prime Minister's Foreword, as 'the most far reaching reform of the National Health Service in its forty year history'. It may indeed, if fully enacted, be just that. One commentator, Robert J. Maxwell, succinctly identified at its core 'an attempt to create within an enormous public service a form of regulated, publicly funded market' (*Observer*, 5 February 1989). As such it does represent a change *vis-à-vis* the NHS before the Griffiths Report (DHSS 1983a). But it must also be seen as consistent with a policy imperative present since then and identified throughout this work. I will comment on four things from the White Paper to underline this point.

The extension of the enterprise culture so exemplified by competitive tendering and privatization and by the introduction of general management is furthered by the proposals to allow opting out by hospitals and the creation of budgets in general practice (Ham 1989, p. 39). The challenge to clinician power and privilege is present in the White Paper in its proposals to introduce managers and management criteria into the award of merit payments. It is not present in the self-regulatory device of Medical Audit. The shift towards central control and a hierarchical health service is present in changes proposed in the personnel of health authorities and particularly the removal of local government nominees. The concentration on a politics of presentation is present in the brevity of the document (and in its 'glossiness'). In the working papers that accompany the White Paper there are just two paragraphs on how hospitals will opt out of their district health authority and not even the most elementary formulations on how drug budgets will be used to control the prescribing practices of GPs (see the editorial in the *Guardian*, 21 January 1989).

If the government had hoped to avoid political criticism and the risk of damage to its aspired status as protector of the NHS then its leaks and its change by stealth did not work. Since the White Paper was made public opposition has been growing. The BMA described the White Paper proposals on opting out as threatening the even spread of medical specialities in the United Kingdom. Perhaps it should have said that they would make worse the uneven spread. The BMA saw the proposals on GP budgets as likely to lead to doctors increasing the size of their lists and offering a worse service to patients. Indeed the BMA Chairman suggested that 'there was very little evidence that much was wrong with the NHS except that it was underfunded' (*Guardian*, 3 March 1989).

I will continue this conclusion by commenting on two areas where there were very real problems for the NHS. One is related to its staffing and specifically to nursing, and the other to the needs of patients, specifically the elderly. Both link with demographic changes now apparent.

Changes in nursing followed considerable debate about the existence and causes of a crisis in nursing. The crisis was seen to be one of both pay and morale and was most vividly exemplified in the rate at which nurses were leaving the profession and the evident immediate and projected future shortage of nurses and midwives. (The Royal College of Midwives complained to the Secretary of State that 17.6 per cent of midwifery posts were unfilled (*Guardian*, 12 February 1988).) But the crisis was also presented as one linked with overall levels of funding of the health authorities. We have seen how nurses' pay increases have repeatedly not been fully funded by the government and consequently, even if pay increases were awarded, they went alongside worsening conditions of work as money was diverted from other health authority projects.

On 21 April 1988 an average pay rise of 15.3 per cent was awarded, with £749 million from the government's contingency reserve being allocated to ensure that health authorities would not have to make compensatory cuts to meet the increase in their payroll. Both the government and many commentators saw the award as something that would 'stem the tide of the health debate' (Guardian, 22 April 1988), a debate in which the government was feeling increasingly beleagured. The pay award was contingent upon a regrading exercise and, consistent with an overall government stance, it seemed to offer inroads for managerial control and pose an attack on professional solidarity. Put simply, it would reward some and then separate higher grades from lower.

Changes in training, known as Project 2000, were welcomed by the Royal College of Nursing as 'the most important development in the profession since Florence Nightingale' (Guardian, 24 May 1988). It was anticipated that the reforms would rationalize nurse training procedures in a standard three-year course; give trainees student status with grants or bursaries rather than salaries; phase out the enrolled nurse grade in favour of a single registered nurse qualification; and cut substantially the workload undertaken by trainees on the wards. The proportion of the nursing workforce that was qualified (currently 59 per cent) would be reduced and a new grade of nurse helper would provide nursing back-up on the ward.

If the pay award and changes in structure were designed to stem the tide of the debate they failed. Three things happened. First, it was argued that the overall allocation to health authorities was not sufficient and so, once more, cuts would have to be made. Second, there was opposition to the divisions the regrading would create between nurses. Third, there were many arguments about the managerial decisions of who should be given higher-grade posts. Indeed the period since April 1988 has been one characterized by considerable anger among nurses and midwives and by widespread industrial action. It remains to be seen if the government's strategic aims will be achieved; their tactical ones have lamentably failed.

A second major area of concern is present in the increase in the number of elderly people in the population. Here two documents provide interesting routes to understanding the interrelationship of policy and need. In 1988 Roy Griffiths (he of the Griffiths Report) reported again (Griffiths 1988). This time his brief was on 'Community Care' and his subtitle was 'Agenda for Action'. That action has not yet been forthcoming. The following year a joint report from the Royal College of

Physicians and the Royal College of Psychiatrists (1989) addressed the care
of the elderly with mental illness.

As we have seen in earlier parts of this work, the elderly make
proportionately more demands on medical services and as the relative and
absolute number of elderly in the population increase the NHS must be
expanded simply to stand still. Community care has been posed as a route
towards a more appropriate service for many in this category. Griffiths
supported the shift of public spending towards more home-based care. He
wanted to simplify relations between local authority and NHS carers and
promote closer working relations between the various agencies involved.
He made a plea that the whole package of community care be adequately
funded. The Royal Colleges would support that plea and put it in the
context of what they identify as a lack of any clear-cut central policy
particularly for the care of the elderly with mental illness. Nationally over
37 per cent of first psychiatric admissions and 33 per cent of readmissions
are of old people.

The care of the elderly is an area where the NHS, local authority and
voluntary sector must work closely together. The danger in an environment that stresses competition, value for money and self-help is
that the planning needed and the level of resource required will not be
made available and a rhetoric of community care will hide a reliance on the
unseen labour of families and friends. As the Royal Colleges (1989, p. 1)
report observes: 'There are few families that do not have some experience
of looking after confused elderly relatives.' This will become more and
more the case and is an area that must be resourced and planned now.

The different parts of the health care system operate using a range of
ideologies, planning imperatives and organizational forms. The system is a
hybrid that requires an analysis that emphasizes the difference between the
parts as much as their interconnections. But overall health policy cannot be
understood unless its totality is grasped.

The NHS arose out of the optimism of post-Second World War Britain
and its founders saw it as part of a movement of social change that would
include full-employment policies, the provision of decent housing, social
insurance and better education. It was the whole prescription and not a
single pill that would effect the cure.

The NHS now operates in an environment where there are around 3
million people out of work; where 16 million are living on, or just above,
the poverty line; and where there has been a sevenfold increase in
homelessness between 1977 and 1987 (*Guardian*, 25 February 1987). It
operates in an environment where, in 1987, nearly 500 people were killed at
work and 178,000 were sufficiently seriously injured to need at least three
days off; and where it is estimated that the actual incidence of injury is
twice the reported rate. The Health and Safety Executive has been cut
back (*Guardian*, 9 March 1988).

It operates in a nation with some of the worst rates of heart illness in the world but where, in 1982, nutrition standards for school meals were abolished; where the government has resisted pressure to curb tobacco advertising further; where the real cost of alcohol is going down; where there is no room in a proposed national curriculum for schools for health and sex education; where sports facilities are being sold off; where there is no agreed formula for labelling food, and where there are still no directors of public health in health authorities (DHSS 1988).

Two quotes to finish will support, I hope, a realization that planning needs to consider totalities and that health policy needs politics – but the politics of change, not of presentation:

Health can't be produced or administered, only allowed or encouraged. Health is the aftertaste of a society's other activities, the residue of all its policies (Karpf 1988; see also the *Guardian*, 11 May 1988).

Finally, Rousseau argues that one facilitates health

not by building hospitals for the poor, but by securing all citizens against poverty (quoted in Berman 1970, p. 209).

Bibliography

Albrow, M.C. (1970). *Bureaucracy.* Macmillan, London.
Allen, D., Harley, M., Makinson, G.T. (1987). 'Performance Indicators in the National Health Service', *Social Policy and Administration*, vol. 21, no. 1, Spring, pp. 70–84.
Allenway, L. (1987). 'A Very Secret Secretariat', *Health Service Journal*, 2 July, pp. 762–3.
Allsop, J. (1984). *Health Policy and the National Health Service.* Longman, London.
Althusser, L. (1977). *For Marx.* New Left Books, London.
Ansoff, H.I. (1965). *Corporate Strategy.* McGraw-Hill, New York.
Arnold, D. (1987). 'Is Management a Common Culture?', *Health Service Journal*, 19 March, p. 332.
Association of Community Health Councils (1988). *Financing the NHS. The Consumer View.* ACHC, 30 Drayton Park, London N5 1PB.
Bailey, J. (1975). *Social Theory for Planning.* Routledge and Kegan Paul, London.
Baly, M.E. (1987). *Florence Nightingale and the Nursing Legacy.* Croom Helm, London.
Basaglia, F. (1981). 'Breaking the Circuit of Control'. In D. Ingleby (ed.), *Critical Psychiatry.* Penguin, Harmondsworth.
Beckett, F. (1984). 'City Bids for Dirty Linen', *New Statesman*, 8 June, p. 14.
Bennis, W.G. (1966). 'Changing Organisations', *Journal of Applied Behavioural Science,* vol. 2, no. 3, pp. 247–63.
Bennis, W.G. (1970). 'The Failure and Promise of the Social Sciences', *Technology Review*, October–November. Reprinted in S.M. Thomas and W.G. Bennis (eds), *Management of Change and Conflict.* Penguin, Harmondsworth, 1972.
Berger, P.L. and Luckman, T. (1966). *The Social Construction of Reality.* Penguin, Harmondsworth.
Berman, M. (1970). *The Politics of Authenticity.* Athenaeum, New York.
Bevan, A. (1952). *In Place of Fear.* William Heinemann, London.
Bion, W.R. (1968). *Experiences in Groups.* Tavistock, London.
Birch, A.H. (1964). *Representative and Responsible Government.* George Allen & Unwin, London.
Blackstone, T. (1979). 'Helping Ministers Do a Better Job', *New Society*, 19 July, pp. 131–2.

Bland, L. (1985). 'Sex and Morals: Rearming the Left', *Marxism Today*, September, pp. 21–4.

Bosanquet, N. (1980). 'Grim Reality', *New Society*, vol. 52, no. 913, 3 April, pp. 17–18.

Boston Women's Health Book Collective (1984). *The New Our Bodies. Ourselves.* Simon and Schuster, New York.

Boyers, R. and Orrill, R. (eds) (1972). *Laing and Anti-Psychiatry.* Penguin, Harmondsworth.

Butts, M., Irving, G. and Whitt, C. (1981). *From Principles to Practice: A Commentary on Health Service Planning and Resource Allocation in England from 1970 to 1980.* Nuffield Provincial Hospitals Trust, London.

Campbell, B. (1987). 'Boy's Own Spies', *Marxism Today*, September, p. 9.

Campbell, R. and Macfarlane, A. (1987). *Where To Be Born?* National Perinatal Epidemiology Unit, Radcliffe Infirmary, Oxford.

Carley, A. (1981). *Social Measurement and Social Indicators.* George Allen & Unwin, London.

Carling, A. (1986). 'Rational Choice Marxism', *New Left Review*, no. 160, November–December, pp. 24–62.

Carrier, J. (1978). 'Positive Discrimination in the Allocation of NHS Resources' in M. Brown and S. Baldwin (eds), *The Yearbook of Social Policy in Britain 1977.* Routledge and Kegan Paul, London, pp. 119–44.

Castle, B. (1976). *N.H.S. Revisited.* Tract no. 440, Fabian Society, London.

Castle, B. (1980). *The Castle Diaries 1974–76.* Weidenfeld and Nicolson, London.

Cawson, A. (1982). *Corporatism and Welfare.* Heinemann, London.

CIPFA (1984). *Health Care U.K. 1984: an Economic, Social and Policy Audit.* Chartered Institute of Public Finance and Administration, London.

Cohen, P. (1984a). 'Dirty Cuts as Hospitals Opt for Private Cleaning', *New Statesman*, 30 March, p. 4.

Cohen, P. (1984b). 'A "Better Class" of Supporter', *New Statesman*, 1 June, p. 6.

Cohen, P. (1986). 'Strange Men Move into NHS', *New Statesman*, 18 April, pp. 13–15.

Cohen, P. and Anderson, G. (1984). 'Mopping Up the Unions', *New Statesman*, 18 May, pp. 12–13.

College of Health (1985). *Guide to Hospital Waiting Lists.* College of Health, 14 Buckingham Street, London WC2N 6DS, College of Health.

College of Health (1987). *Guide to the Waiting Lists 1987.* College of Health, London.

Collingwood, R.G. (1924). *The Map of Knowledge.* Oxford University Press, Oxford.

Comptroller and Auditor General (1985). *Control of Nursing Manpower. National Audit Office Report.* HMSO, London.

Conservative Party (1979). *The Conservative Manifesto.* Conservative Central Office, London.

Conservative Party (1987). *The Next Moves Forward.* Conservative Central Office, London.

Cooper, M.H. (1975). *Rationing Health Care.* Croom Helm, London.

Crossman, R. (1977). *The Diaries of a Cabinet Minister, Vol 3.* Hamish Hamilton/ Jonathan Cape, London.

Crozier, M. (1964). *The Bureaucratic Phenomenon*. Tavistock, London.

Dahl, R.A. (1961). *Who Governs?* Yale University Press, New Haven, CT.

Dahl, R.A. and Lindblom, C.E. (1953). *Politics, Economics and Welfare*. Harper and Row, New York.

Dahrendorf, R. (1959). *Class and Class Conflict in Industrial Society*. Routledge and Kegan Paul, London.

Davey, B. (1988). 'Social Side of Cancer', *Marxism Today*, March, pp. 30–3.

Davidson, N. (1987). *A Question of Care: The Changing Face of the National Health Service*. Michael Joseph, London.

Department of Health (1989). *Working for Patients*, Cm 555. HMSO, London.

Department of Health and Social Security (1969). *Report of the Committee of Inquiry into Allegations of Ill-treatment of Patients and Other Irregularities at the Ely Hospital, Cardiff*, Cmnd 3957. HMSO, London.

DHSS (1972). DHSS. *National Health Service Reorganisation: England*, Cmnd 5055. HMSO, London.

DHSS (1974). *Management Arrangements for the Reorganised National Health Service*. HMSO, London.

DHSS (1976a). *Sharing Resources for Health in England. Report of the Resource Allocation Working Party*. HMSO, London.

DHSS (1976b). *Fit for the Future. Report of the Committee on Child Health Services* (Court Report). HMSO, London.

DHSS (1981). *Orthopaedic Services: Waiting Time for Out-patient Appointments and In-patient Treatment* (Duthie Report). HMSO, London.

DHSS (1983a). *NHS Management Inquiry* (Griffiths Report). HMSO, London.

DHSS (1983b). *Revised Pharmaceutical Price Regulation Scheme*, Press Notice 83/276, 8 December.

DHSS (1984a). *The Health Service in England. Annual Report*. HMSO, London.

DHSS (1984b). *Public Expenditure on the Social Services*, Cmnd 9414, HMSO, London.

DHSS (1984c). *Minister Acts to Curb Exceptionally Favourable Prices for Drugs*, Press Notice 847358, 13 November.

DHSS (1985). *Reform of Social Security*. Cmnd 9517, 9518, 9519. HMSO, London.

DHSS (1986a). *Public Expenditure on the Social Services. Response by the Government to the Fourth Report from the Social Services Committee, Session 1985–86*, Cm 27. HMSO, London.

DHSS (1986b). *Review of the RAWP Formula* (Letter from the Chairman of the NHS Management Board, Victor Paige, to Consultants).

DHSS (1986c). *Management of Private Practice in Health Service Hospitals*. HMSO, London.

DHSS (1988). *Public Health in England: The Report of the Committee of Inquiry into the Future Development of the Public Health Function (Chairman Sir Donald Acheson)*, Cm 289. HMSO, London.

Doyal, L. and Pennell, I. (1979). *The Political Economy of Health*. Pluto Press, London.

Doyal, L. (1983a). *Cancer in Britain*. Pluto Press, London.

Doyal, L. (1983b). 'Women, Health and the Sexual Division of Labour: A Case Study of the Women's Health Movement in Britain', *Critical Social Policy*, vol. 7, Summer, pp. 21–33.

Dunnell, K. and Holland, W.W. (1973). 'Planning for Health Services' in *Annual*

Report: St Thomas's Social Medicine and Health Services Research Unit. St Thomas's Hospital and Medical School, London.

Escudero, J.C. (1980). 'Starting from Year One: The Politics of Health in Nicaragua', *International Journal of Health Services*, vol. 10, no. 4, pp. 647–56.

Eversley, D. (1975). *Planning Without Growth.* Fabian Research Series 321. Fabian Society, London.

Finch, J. and Groves, D. (1986). *Labour of Love: Women, Work and Caring.* Routledge and Kegan Paul, London.

Florey, C. du V. and Weddell, J.M. (1976). 'The Epidemiologists' Contribution' in K. Dunnell (ed.), *Health Service Planning.* King Edward's Hospital Fund, London.

Foot, M. (1975). *Aneurin Bevan, Vol. 2: 1945–60.* Paladin, St Albans.

Frolich, P. (1983). *Rosa Luxemburg.* Pluto Press, London.

Gabbay, J. and Dopson, S. (1987). 'The Search for a Shared Vision' *Health and Social Services Journal* 10 September, pp. 1042–3.

Goodin, R.E. (1982). 'Rational Politicians and Rational Bureaucrats in Washington and Whitehall', *Public Administration*, vol. 60, no. 1, pp. 23–41.

Gough, I. (1979). *The Political Economy of the Welfare State.* Macmillan, London.

Grey-Turner, E. and Sutherland, F.M. (1982). *History of the British Medical Association 1932–1981.* BMA, London.

Griffiths, R. (1988). *Community Care: Agenda for Action: A Report to the Secretary of State for Social Services.* HMSO, London.

Guillebaud, C.W. (1956). *Report of the Committee of Inquiry into the Cost of the National Health Service*, Cmd 9663. HMSO, London.

Habermas, J. (1979). *Communication and the Evolution of Society.* Heinemann, London.

Hall, S. and Jacques, M. (1983). *The Politics of Thatcherism.* Lawrence and Wishart, London.

Halpern, S. (1985). 'How Should the Centre Be Spread?', *Health and Social Services Journal*, 28 February, pp. 248–50.

Ham, C.J. (1981). *Policy Making in the National Health Service.* Macmillan, London.

Ham, C. (1985). *Health Policy in Britain*, 2nd edn. Macmillan, London.

Ham, C. (1989). 'Clarke's Strong Medicine', *Marxism Today*, March, pp. 38–41.

Harvey-Jones, J. (1988). *Making It Happen.* Collins, London.

Hayek, F.A. von (1944). *The Road to Serfdom.* Routledge, London.

Health Education Council (1987). *The Health Divide: Inequalities in Health in the 1980s.* HEC, London.

Hearn, J. (1982). 'Decrementalism: The Practice of Cuts and the Theory of Planning' in P. Healey, G. McDougall and M.J. Thomas (eds), *Planning Theory: Prospects for the 1980s.* Pergamon, Oxford.

Hearn, J. and Roberts, I. (1975). 'Planning under Difficulties: The Move to Decrementalism' in K. Jones and S. Baldwin (eds), *The Yearbook of Social Policy in Britain 1975.* Routledge and Kegan Paul, London.

Hearn, J. and Small, N. (1984). 'Planning the Personal Social Services' in C. Jones and J. Stevenson (eds), *The Year Book of Social Policy in Britain 1983.* Routledge and Kegan Paul, London.

Heydebrand, W. (1980). 'Organisational Contradictions in Public Bureaucracy: Towards a Marxian Theory of Organisations' in A. Etzioni and E.W.

Lehman (eds), *A Sociological Reader in Complex Organisations*. Holt Reinhart, London.

Hinshelwood, R. and Manning, N. (eds) (1979). *Therapeutic Communities: Reflections and Progress*. Routledge and Kegan Paul, London.

Hobsbawm, E. (1987). 'Out of the Wilderness', *Marxism Today*, October, pp. 12–19.

Hospitals and Health Services Commission (1974). *A Report on Hospitals in Australia*. Australian Government Publishing Service, Canberra.

House of Commons (1972). *National Health Service Reorganisation: England*, Cmnd 5055, HMSO, London.

House of Commons Committee of Public Accounts (1981). *17th Report: Financial Control and Accountability in the National Health Service*, Session 1980–1, HC 255. HMSO, London.

House of Commons Committee of Public Accounts (1986a). *14th Report: Control of Nursing Manpower*, Session 1985–6, HC 98. HMSO, London.

House of Commons Committee of Public Accounts (1986b). *42nd Report: Value for Money Developments in the National Health Service: Energy Conservation*, Session 1985–6, HC 335. HMSO, London.

House of Commons Committee of Public Accounts (1986c). *12th Report: British Oxygen Company and the National Health Service*, Session 1985–6, HC 67.

House of Commons Committee of Public Accounts (1987). *8th Report: Financial Reporting to Parliament*, Session 1986–7, HC 98.

House of Commons Committee of Public Accounts (1988a). *11th Report: Internal Audit in the National Health Service*, Session 1987–8, HC 156.

House of Commons Committee of Public Accounts (1988b). *Estate Management in the National Health Service*, Session 1987–8, HC 481.

House of Commons Social Services Committee (1984). *Griffiths NHS Management Inquiry Report. First Report from the Social Services Committee*, Session 1983–4, HC 209. HMSO, London.

House of Commons Social Services Committee (1986). *4th Report: Public Expenditure on the Social Services*, Session 1985–6, HC 387–I/II. HMSO, London.

House of Commons Trade and Industry Committee (1973). *Monopolies Commission Report*, Session 1972–3, HC 268, vol. 12.

Hunter, D.J. (1980). *Coping with Uncertainty. Policy and Politics in the NHS*. Research Studies Press, Chichester.

Iliffe, S. (1983). *The NHS. A Picture of Health?* Lawrence and Wishart, London.

Illich, I. (1977). *Limits to Medicine*. Penguin, Harmondsworth.

Ingle, S. and Tether, P. (1981). *Parliament and Health Policy: The Role of MPs, 1970–5*. Gower, Aldershot.

Institute of Economic Affairs (1987). *Medicines in the Market Place*. IEA Health Unit, 2 Lord North Street, London SW1.

Iverson, S. (1984). 'A Private Way to Stop Kidney Deaths', *New Statesman*, 4 May, p. 2.

Jackson, P.M. (1982). *The Political Economy of Bureaucracy*. Philip Allan, Oxford.

Karpf, A. (1988). *Doctoring the Media: The Reporting of Health and Medicine*. Routledge, London.

Kemp, R. (1982). 'Critical Planning Theory—Review and Critique' in P. Healey,

G. McDougall and M.J. Thomas (eds), *Planning Theory: Prospects for the 1980s*. Pergamon, Oxford.

King's Fund Institute (1987a). *Public Expenditure and the NHS: Trends and Prospects*. King's Fund Institute, 126 Albert Street, London NW1.

King's Fund Institute (1987b). *Planned Health Services for Inner London*. King's Fund Institute, London.

Labour Party (1987). *Britain Will Win*. Labour Party, London.

Land, H. and Rose, H. (1986). 'Compulsory Altruism for Some. Or An Altruistic Society for All' in P. Bean, J. Ferris and D. Whyness (eds), *In Defence of Welfare*. Tavistock, London.

Le Fanu, J. (1985). 'Doctors dilemma', *New Statesman*, 1 February, p. 12.

Lichtner, S. and Pflanz, M. (1971). 'Appendectomy in the Federal Republic of Germany: Epidemiology and Medical Care Patterns', *Medical Care*, ix, 311.

Lindblom, C.E. (1964). 'The Science of Muddling Through' in H.J. Leavitt and L.R. Pondy (eds), *Readings in Managerial Psychology*. University of Chicago Press, Chicago.

Lloyd, J. (1986). 'Busy Izzy in Search of Truth', *New Statesman*, 15 August, pp. 18–19.

London Health Emergency (1986). *Hitting the Skids: a Catalogue of NHS Cuts in London*. London Health Emergency, London.

Lovell, A.M. (1978). 'From Confinement to Community: The Radical Transformation of an Italian Mental Hospital', *State and Mind*. vol. 6, no. 3, pp. 7–11.

Lukács, G. (1971). *History and Class Consciousness*. Merlin, London.

Lukes, S. (1974). *Power: a Radical View*. Macmillan, London.

Margolis, J. (1975). Comment. *Journal of Law and Economics*, vol. 18, pp. 645–59.

Marshall, G. (1981). 'Accounting for Deviance', *International Journal of Sociology and Social Policy*, vol. 1, no. 1.

Maternity Services Advisory Committee (1985). *Maternity Care in Action*. HMSO, London.

Maynard, A. (1986). 'Policy Choices in the Health Sector', in R. Berthoud (ed.), *Challenges to Social Policy*. Policy Studies Institute, London.

Mays, N. and Bevan, G. (1987). *Resource Allocation in the Health Service*. Bedford Square Press, London.

McKeown, T. (1979). *The Role of Medicine*. Basil Blackwell, Oxford.

McLuhan, M. (1964). *Understanding Media*. Sphere, London.

Medical Services Review Committee (1962). *A Review of the Medical Services in Great Britain* (Porritt Report). HMSO, London.

Menzies, I.E.P. (1960). 'A Case Study in the Functioning of Social Systems as a Defence against Anxiety', *Human Relations*, vol. 13, no. 2, May, pp. 95–121.

Merton, R.K. (1957). *Social Theory and Social Structure*. Free Press, New York.

Ministry of Health (1951). *Report for 1949–50, Part II, On the State of the Public Health* (Annual Report of the Chief Medical Officer), Cmd 8343. HMSO, London.

Ministry of Health (1952). *Report of the Ministry of Health Covering the Period April 1, 1950 to Dec. 31, 1951*, Cmd 8655. HMSO, London.

Ministry of Health (1957). *Report of the Ministry of Health for the Year Ending Dec. 31, 1956*, Cmnd 293. HMSO, London.

Ministry of Health (1962). *A Hospital Plan for England and Wales*, Cmnd 1604. HMSO, London.

Ministry of Health (1966). *Report of the Committee on Senior Nursing Staff Structure (Chairman Brian Salmon)*. HMSO, London.

Ministry of Health (1967). *First Report of the Joint Working Party on the Organisation of Medical Work in Hospitals* (Cogwheel Report), HMSO, London. Subsequent Reports by the Working Party were in 1972 and 1974 and were made under the aegis of the Department of Health and Social Security.

Monopolies and Restrictive Practices Commission (1957). *Supply of Certain Industrial and Medical Gases*, Session 1956–7, I–IC 13.

Moore, W. (1970). 'Changes in American Social Structure', *Denver Law Review*, vol. 44, Fall. Reprinted in J.M. Thomas and W.G. Bennis (eds), *Management of Change and Conflict*. Penguin, Harmondsworth, 1972.

Mulkay, M., Ashmore, M. and Pinch, T. (1987). 'Measuring the Quality of Life: A Sociological Invention Concerning the Application of Economics to Health Care', *Sociology*, vol. 21, no. 4, November, pp. 541–64.

National Audit Office (1987). *Competitive Tendering for Support Services in the National Health Service. Report by the Comptroller and Auditor General*, Session 1986–7, HC 318. HMSO, London.

National Association of Health Authorities (1987). *Cross-Boundary Patient Flows*. Garth House, Birmingham.

National Children's Bureau (1987). *Investing in the Future*. NCB, 8 Wakley Place, London EC1V 7QE.

Neale, J. (1983). *Memories of a Callous Picket*. Pluto, London.

NHS Unlimited (1986). Report c/o Frank Dobson MP, House of Commons, Westminster, London SW1.

Nickson, R. (1985). 'Dawn of the age of accountability', *Health and Social Service Journal*, Jan 10, pp. 41–3.

Nisbet, R. (1969). *Social Change and History: Aspects of the Western Theory of Development*. Oxford University Press, Oxford.

Niskanen, W. (1973). *Bureaucracy and Representative Government*. Aldine-Atherton, New York.

Nutbeam, D. and Catford, J. (1987). *Pulse of Wales Social Survey. Heartbeat Report*. Cardiff Directorate of the Welsh Heart Programme.

Oakley, A. and Graham, H. (1982). 'Competing Ideologies of Reproduction' in H. Roberts (ed.), *Women, Health and Reproduction*. Routledge and Kegan Paul, London.

Office of Health Economics (1984). *Compendium of Health Statistics 1985*. OHE, 12 Whitehall, London SW1.

Office of Health Economics (1987). *Compendium of Health Statistics 1987*. OHE, London.

Office of Population Censuses and Surveys (1986). *Occupational Mortality. The Registrar General's Decennial Supplement for Great Britain 1979–80, 1982–83*. HMSO, London.

O'Higgins, M. (1987). *Health Spending—A Way to Sustainable Growth*. Institute of Health Services Management, London.

Owen, D. (1976). *In Sickness and in Health*. Quartet Books, London.

Parston, G. (1980). *Planners, Politics and Health Services*. Croom Helm, London.

People's Campaign for Health, c/o 46 Blayton Road, Sheffield S4 7DH.

Philips, M. (1965). *Small Social Groups in England*. Methuen, London.
Porter, M. (1987). 'Corporate Strategy. The State of Strategic Thinking', *The Economist*, 23 May, pp. 21–8.
Powell, E. (1966). *A New Look at Medicine and Politics*. Pitman Medical, London.
Radical Statistics Health Group (1980). *The Unofficial Guide to Official Health Statistics*. British Society for Social Responsibility in Science, London.
Radical Statistics Health Group (1985). *Unsafe in their Hands*. British Society for Social Responsibility in Science, London.
Radical Statistics Health Group (1987). *Facing the Figures*. British Society for Social Responsibility in Science, London.
Rahman, N. (1987). *Nursing a Grievance: Low Pay in Nursing*. Low Pay Unit, London.
Rentoul, J. and Cohen, P. (1984). 'Beyond the "Reverse the Cuts" slogans', *New Statesman*, 10 February, p. 8.
Richardson, J.J. and Jordan, A.G. (1979). *Governing under Pressure: The Policy Process in a Post-Parliamentary Democracy*. Martin Robertson, Oxford.
Rodmell, S. and Watt, A. (eds) (1986). *The Politics of Health Education*. Routledge and Kegan Paul, London.
Roth, A. (1970). *Enoch Powell: Tory Tribune*. Macdonald, London.
Roy, D.H. (1968). 'The Union-Organizing Campaign as a Problem of Social Distance: Three Crucial Dimensions of Affiliation–Disaffiliation', in H.S. Becker *et al.* (eds), *Institutions and the Person*. Aldine, New York.
Royal College of Physicians and Royal College of Psychiatrists (1989). *Care of Elderly People with Mental Illness*. Royal College of Physicians/Royal College of Psychiatrists, London.
Said, E. (1978). *Orientalism*. Penguin, Harmondsworth.
Said, E. (1986). 'On Palestinian Identity: A Conversation with Salman Rushdie', *New Left Review*, no. 160, November–December, pp. 63–80.
Savage, W. (1986). *A Savage Enquiry. Who Controls Childbirth?* Virago, London.
Self, P. (1977). *Administrative Theories and Politics*, 2nd edn. George Allen & Unwin, London.
Skeet, M. (1978). 'The Experience of the Third World' in M. Skeet and K. Elliott (eds), *Health Auxiliaries and the Health Team*. Croom Helm, London.
Small, N. (1987). 'Putting Violence to Social Workers into Context', *Critical Social Policy*, no. 19, Summer, pp. 40–51.
Small, N. (1988). 'Aids and Social Policy', *Critical Social Policy*, no. 21, Spring, pp. 9–29.
Smith, G. and Cantley, C. (1985). *Assessing Health Care*. Open University Press, Milton Keynes.
Social Democratic Party (1987). *The Alliance for Health*. SDP, 4 Cowley Street, London SW1.
Social Democratic Party, Liberal Alliance (1987). *Britain United. The Time Has Come*. SDP, Liberal Alliance, London.
Stanyer, J. and Smith, B. (1976). *Administering Britain*. Fontana, London.
Sutherland, I. (1987). *Health Education—Half a Policy: The Rise and Fall of the Health Education Council*. National Extension College, Cambridge.
Teeling-Smith, G. (ed.) (1987). *Health Economics: Prospects for the Future*. Croom Helm, London.

Thane, P. (1982). *Foundations of the Welfare State*. Longman, London.

Thrasher, M. (1984). 'The Role of Administrative Discretion in Public Sector Organisations', paper presented to British Sociological Association Conference 'Work, Employment and Unemployment', Bradford University, 2–5 April.

Thunhurst, C. (1985–6). 'Close Encounters of an Economic Kind', *Radical Community Medicine*, Winter, pp. 18–26.

Touraine, A. (1974). *The Post-industrial Society*. London, Wildwood House.

Touraine, A. (1983). *Solidarity*. Cambridge University Press, Cambridge.

Townsend, P. and Davidson, N. (eds) (1982). *Inequalities in Health. The Black Report*. Penguin, Harmondsworth.

Turner, B.S. (1987). *Medical Power and Social Knowledge*. Sage, London.

Underwood, J. (1976). 'Structural Explanations of Planners' Use of Theory in Practice', mimeo, Central London Polytechnic.

Wainwright, H. (1987). 'Beyond Labourism', *New Left Review*, no. 164, July–August, pp. 34–51.

Wallis, R. and Bruce, S. (1983). 'Accounting for Action: Defending the Common Sense Heresy', *Sociology*, vol. 17, no. 1, February, pp. 97–111.

Watkins, S. (1987). *Medicine and Labour. The Politics of a Profession*. Lawrence and Wishart, London.

Webb, A. and Wistow, G. (1982). *Whither State Welfare?* Royal Institute of Public Administration, London.

Weber, M. (1948). *From Max Weber: Essays in Sociology*. H.H. Gerth and C. Wright Mills, (eds). Routledge and Kegan Paul, London.

Weber, M. (1949). *The Methodology of the Social Sciences*. Free Press, Glencoe, IL.

Werner, D. (1978). 'The Village Health Worker: Lackey or Liberator?' in M. Skeet and K. Elliott (eds), *Health Auxiliaries and the Health Team*. Croom Helm, London.

West of Scotland Politics of Health Group (1984). *Glasgow: Health of a City*. West of Scotland Politics of Health Group, Glasgow.

Which? (1984). 'Private Medical Insurance', June, pp. 256–64.

Widgery, D. (1979). *Health in Danger*. Macmillan, London.

Wildavsky, A. (1964). *The Politics of the Budgetary Process*. Little Brown, Boston.

Williams, A. (1985). 'Economics of Coronary Artery Bypass Grafting', *British Medical Journal*, vol. 291, pp. 326–9.

Williams, A. (1987). 'Measuring Quality of Life: A Comment', *Sociology*, vol. 21, no. 4, November, pp. 565–6.

Wrapp, H.E. (1967). 'Good Managers Don't Make Policy Decisions', *Harvard Business Review*, September–October, pp. 91–6.

Yates, J. (1987). *Why Are We Waiting? An Analysis of Hospital Waiting Lists*. Oxford University Press, Oxford.

Young, K. (1977). 'Values in the Policy Process', *Policy and Politics*, vol. 5, no. 3, pp. 1–24.

Index